VALUES, ETHICS AND HEALTH CARE

VALUES, ETHICS AND HEALTH CARE

PETER DUNCAN

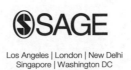

Los Angeles | London | New Delhi
Singapore | Washington DC

First published 2010

SAGE Publications Ltd
1 Oliver's Yard
55 City Road
London EC1Y 1SP

SAGE Publications Inc.
2455 Teller Road
Thousand Oaks, California 91320

SAGE Publications India Pvt Ltd
B 1/I 1 Mohan Cooperative Industrial Area
Mathura Road, Post Bag 7
New Delhi 110 044

SAGE Publications Asia-Pacific Pte Ltd
33 Pekin Street #02-01
Far East Square
Singapore 048763

Library of Congress Control Number: 2008941744

British Library Cataloguing in Publication data

A catalogue record for this book is available from
the British Library

ISBN 978-1-4129-2351-4
ISBN 978-1-4129-2352-1 (pbk)

Typeset by C&M Digitals (P) Ltd, Chennai, India
Printed in Great Britain by the MPG Books Group
Printed on paper from sustainable resources

CONTENTS

ACKNOWLEDGEMENTS

I would like to thank my colleagues in the Department of Education and Professional Studies, King's College London, for their continued support. Once more I am especially grateful to Alan Cribb and Margaret Sills for helping me to organise a period of study leave during which I was able to think a lot about the subject matter of this book, and ultimately to write a significant part of it.

Zoe Elliott-Fawcett and her colleagues at Sage have been a great help, right from the stage where the initial ideas for this project developed.

I am grateful to the anonymous reviewers of both the original proposal and the draft manuscript for their very useful advice and comments.

The students with whom I have worked over the last few years at King's College London have helped me greatly, not least by constantly reminding me through our discussions of the ambiguity and difficulty that is almost always inherent in the practice of health care. Their experience, and the examples that they have helped to generate, have been central in allowing me to understand what I have come to call 'ordinary' health care as in actual fact being quite *extraordinary*.

Finally, and most importantly, I would like to thank Jane for all the support she gives me, in all kinds of different ways.

PREFACE

This book rests on the broad but essential claim that the whole enterprise of health care is fundamentally to do with values and ethics. Unless we have a concern with questions of ethics and values, our conception of health care, and our interest in practice, is incomplete. This claim is not in any sense a new one. Indeed, part of this book's project is to do with charting the history of the claim, and how (as well as why) arguments have been developed to support it.

In the context of the powerful and exciting history of values and ethics in health care, I am trying in this book to do a number of particular things, which I want briefly to outline at its beginning before actually attempting to do them.

First, I am trying to explore the nature of values in the health care context. I am particularly interested in two things here. One is the nature of the value of health itself. Given that one of our working assumptions about health care might be that its purpose is to produce more 'health', we are often remarkably unclear about what we may mean by this. If the purpose of health care is 'more health', yet we are not quite sure of what we understand by that, we lay ourselves open to confusion, dispute (with others who possess alternative understandings) and ultimately dilemmas of ethics in our practice. The history of dispute about the nature of health is probably as good a demonstration as any that we will never be able to reach harmonious agreement about the nature of health as a value. However, if we side-step it altogether, we run the very real risk of being unable to progress very far at all in our explorations of values and ethics in the health care context. So it forms an essential first step in this book, along with my other interest at this point – how and why we develop the health and health care-related values that we actually have. My own view is that they develop in large part through our working, or training to work, in health care, and if this is so, such an idea has major implications for our beliefs and judgements about what we should be doing and why we should be doing it.

The second thing I am trying to do is to understand these values that develop in and from our health care *persona* and practice as drivers of work and ethics in the field. My interest here is largely (although not entirely) in what throughout this book I will call 'ordinary' health care. This is the everyday practice that those working, or training to work, in health care are most likely to be involved in. It includes things like giving advice, arranging care, supporting people trying to change their health behaviour, and so on. There are two reasons for my focus on the ethics of 'ordinary' health care. The first reason, obviously, is that this is the kind of practice most health care workers will be involved with most of the time – and which, at least on occasions, is perhaps thought of as being routine and not worth submitting to ethical examination. Second, against this possible thought, I want to claim that the 'ordinary' in health care is very often quite *extra-ordinary*. If we think of the apparently simple act of giving advice to a patient, say, there are so many layers to consider: her beliefs, values and attitudes as well as our own; the institutional context in which the advice-giving takes place; the social context framing it all, and so on. This is what makes 'ordinary' health care so extraordinary and, in my view, so difficult to deliberate upon. When I talk of 'ordinary' health care, then, I am not in any sense doing so pejoratively.

In this focus on 'ordinary' health care, my intention is not to deliberately exclude what many people might actually more often see as 'extraordinary' health care situations – 'life and death' problems such as abortion, euthanasia, genetic engineering, and so on. Indeed, my argument in support of a fundamental concern for values and ethics in health care begins in part with a study of the particular 'extraordinary' health care situation of assisted suicide. Clearly, there is an essential social need to discuss and deliberate on 'life and death' in health care. But for the reasons I have given above, this is not my main intention here.

The third particular thing that this book tries to do is to cast a concern with values and ethics in health care as one that is (or should be) shared across occupations and professions. This is a book about values and ethics in *health care*, not in nursing or occupational therapy or health-related social work or any other particular health care occupation. Again, there are reasons for this. I want to demonstrate that the values and ethics-related 'agenda' in health care is a shared one. It seems especially important to do this at a time when there is much focus on interdisciplinary and multidisciplinary learning and political attempts are being made (rightly or wrongly) to break down professional barriers. Of course, throughout the book I will be using examples that draw on particular professional contexts or experiences – those of nursing, say. This is because, for better or worse, we tend to organise and understand the world of health care through professional and occupational divisions of one sort or another. But the claim and argument of this book is that there is much more for us to share (occupationally and professionally) with regard to values and ethics in health care than there is to divide.

In attempting to do these things, there is also at least one thing that I am trying to avoid. I want to avoid this book becoming a one-sided explication of theory, or of problems in practice. In one sense, I suppose that somebody could argue that it has to be so. After all, I am writing and you are reading. I am deciding on direction and you are following. But in an important way my intention is for the book to be as unlike this as possible. Throughout the text there are questions, points for thought and examples that are my attempt to engage in shared *dialogue and thinking* with you, albeit within the constraint and limits of the writer–reader divide. But my effort towards establishing a dialogue is a genuine one because I believe that the questions I am posing, the thoughts I am trying to stimulate and the reasoning and reflection I am trying to encourage, is not the writer's responsibility alone. Progress in trying to understand the questions and difficulties that we will discuss has to be shared simply because it cannot be made by oneself.

What I hope to come up with in this book are some possible ways of starting to think about questions of values and ethics in health care. These might be thought of as *frameworks* within which debate can take place. My intention is to try to encourage you to work with my frameworks, or to begin to develop your own conceptions of what is required to try to understand problems in this area. What I am doing, if you like, is to supply some scaffolding poles and planks and start to put them up in a particular way so that they fit my understanding of what needs to be built. But you might want to bring along more or different poles and planks, or rearrange the ones that we already have, to fit your own understanding.

A few final clarifications are needed. First, at certain places in the text I have put words or phrases into **bold** type to indicate that this is a key term or topic under consideration at that point of the book. Second, as I suggested above, the 'Q' (Question) and 'Thinking About…' features are both intended to promote shared dialogue and thinking. However, within this broad intention they have different purposes. 'Q' features ask you to apply yourself to a particular question raised by the text, which I then generally go on to explore in what follows. 'Thinking About…' features are intended to provoke wider reflection, perhaps moving beyond the boundaries of the text itself. Third, the book begins with a series of case studies and continues right the way through with examples that in turn are provided to support thinking, discussion and questioning. The case studies are all taken from 'real life'. This is also true of most of the examples, as they have been generated through discussions with students and colleagues, with whom I have been involved over a number of years, about their own experiences of working in or studying health care and its practices. (I have anonymised examples as appropriate.) For this particularly, I would like to re-iterate the thanks I offered to all these people in my earlier acknowledgements.

HEALTH CARE: WHY SHOULD WE BE CONCERNED ABOUT VALUES AND ETHICS?

Learning Outcomes

By the end of this chapter, you should be able to:

o Identify and discuss a range of health care situations in which consideration of values and ethics is important;
o Critically appraise the worth of the view that a concern with values and ethics is an essential requirement for all those involved in health care;
o Begin a personal account and justification of the importance of values and ethics to your own practice, or study.

Introduction

I am beginning this book with a claim. My claim is that everyone involved in health care should have a fundamental concern with issues of values and ethics. Whatever your occupation, regardless of the activity you are engaged in, the nature and practice of health care demands this concern. From the midwife running an antenatal class through to the nurse caring for a terminally ill patient, from the health promotion specialist planning a smoking prevention programme for young people through to the occupational therapist assessing an elderly person's ability to cope in their own home, this concern is essential. Indeed, I would want to extend my claim further. I would want to say that unless we actually have this fundamental concern with ethics and values as part of our health care-related thinking and practice, we can't properly see ourselves as engaged in health care at all.

Q.:At the very beginning of this book, do you agree with the first part of my claim – that everyone involved in health care, regardless of their occupation, or the activity they are involved in, should have a concern with values and ethics? Do you agree with the second part – that unless we have this concern, we are not properly engaged in health care at all? Whether you agree with me or not, *why* do you hold the view that you have? Make a written note of your responses to these questions and refer to it as you work your way through the rest of this chapter, and other parts of the book, to see if your initial position, and your justification for it, might be changing.

This claim – that we should each have a concern with values and ethics in all of our activities, and that unless we do so we are not properly engaged in health care at all – is a large one to be making. It's possible that you may completely disagree with one or both parts of it. One response to the question I posed above might have been: I just get on with my job as best as I can so why do I need to think about values and ethics? Perhaps more likely, you may agree that some aspects of health care involve difficult questions of ethics (whether and when we should deliberately end life, for example), but that most day-to-day practice requires nothing more than honesty and good intentions. So even if you accept the first part of the claim, you might be very doubtful about the second part. Surely, doing your best is good enough, at least for most of the time?

In some ways, this is a realistic and reasonable response. Those involved in health care practice, whatever their occupation, are busy people. They are often trying to deal with others who are in very difficult circumstances. They are frequently doing so with limited resources. We might well view the seemingly esoteric concerns of ethics as being of little relevance in these kinds of situations (Seedhouse, 1998). Surely, the rubric of 'doing your best' is the one that counts the most here?

I want to argue, though, that while this kind of response is understandable, it is not sufficient. It is not sufficient for two reasons. First, *what exactly* do we mean by 'doing your best'? What counts as 'best'? Who decides what this is? One answer to this last question is to say that it is up to individual practitioners. But if that is so, we are leaving an awful lot up to these individuals. Are we *really* happy to suggest to the individual midwife or nurse, the health promotion specialist or the occupational therapist, that how they decide to conduct their practice, and what counts as '*best* practice' is entirely down to them? This seems to be both unfair to patients or clients, and an unacceptable weight on health care professionals themselves.

The second reason why the response of 'doing your best' is not sufficient is because even if health care practitioners were able (or wanted to) establish what exactly this meant by themselves, there would be a potentially infinite variety of situations in which they would have to apply this rule. (This is accepting in the first place the idea that 'doing your best' is enough of a rule to provide a guide to your action.) What does 'doing your best' mean for the midwife working with an antenatal class? What does it mean for the occupational therapist undertaking a home assessment for an elderly person? The difficulty now is that not only do we potentially have practitioners who might be ambivalent about their capacity to apply a rule, but we also face a range of situations in which that rule might be applied.

It is all beginning to look a little like peeling the skin off an onion. We think about one question, then another appears, and then another. Posing rigorous and appropriate questions is, of course, an important part of academic work (Bonnett, 2001). The kinds of questions that I've just raised are in response to views some might express about the lack of, or limits to, the use in thinking about values and ethics in health care. But simply asking questions is not enough here. There is a need for me to *justify* my initial claim that everyone involved in health care, regardless of what they are doing, should have a concern with values and ethics and that unless this is present, we can't consider someone to be properly engaged in health care at all. Part of this justification must involve thinking carefully about the nature of values, and of ethics. This is a task that I will undertake a little later. At the moment, I want to concentrate on the idea that questions of values and ethics emerge in all aspects and contexts of health care.

To do this, I'm going to examine three separate 'case studies'. The studies are quite different from each other. They have been deliberately chosen to be different because my intention is to demonstrate that values and ethics permeate the entire field of health care. If I can show that ethics and values-related difficulties emerge in contrasting parts of the field, my claim that all health care workers engaged in any kind of activity or intervention should be concerned with them will be supported. It will then be possible to move on to more detailed discussion about the nature of values and ethics, and how they connect with practice and policy in health care. It will also be *easier* to do so because doubts about the worth of a project looking at values and ethics – 'What has all this got to do with *me*?' – will have been addressed.

Thinking About...

As you read through the following case studies, consider carefully whether they bear any similarity to aspects of your own experience. If they do, identify that experience, how you think and feel about it now, and if possible how you thought and felt about it at the time that it happened. If you cannot find any similarity in any of the studies, consider why you believe that to be the case.

Case Study: Living and Dying

Let's start by thinking about the kind of case where many people (possibly) might see ethics and values-based discussion as being important, and as playing an essential part in deciding what to do (or at least in deciding how we feel about and react to what is done).

In August 2005, retired GP Michael Irwin travelled with 74-year-old widow May Murphy from Glasgow to Zurich in Switzerland. Mrs Murphy, who was terminally ill, intended to kill herself with the support of the Zurich-based organisation Dignitas, which helps terminally ill people end their lives (Dyer, 2006). In the apartment used by the organisation, Mrs Murphy took a lethal dose of barbiturates. Dr Irwin was present in the room with Mrs Murphy and her younger son Alan when she swallowed the barbiturate solution:

> He [Dr Irwin] recalls her saying, 'I want to die, my body has gone' ... 'She could hardly move her arms. She had to use both hands in order to hold this little glass,' he said. (Dyer, 2006)

Assisted suicide is against the law in the United Kingdom, so Mrs Murphy and Dr Irwin had travelled to Switzerland, where the practice is legal. But some months after his return to England, Surrey police interviewed him under caution about his role in Mrs Murphy's death. In January 2006, the Crown Prosecution Service was actively considering a possible prosecution of the doctor after he had admitted helping a number of people to receive support from Dignitas.

The issue of assisted suicide is deeply contentious and controversial. A bill to permit it under certain circumstances, introduced into the House of Lords by Lord Joffe, was blocked in May 2006 by a majority of his peers. The bill, based on practice in the state of Oregon in the USA, would have given doctors the right to preside over the administration of lethal drugs to a patient. The patient would be able to request such drugs if his death within six months was certain, and if he was mentally competent and suffering unbearable pain (Woodward, 2006). In the debate that preceded the Lords' rejection, Lord Joffe said:

> As a caring society we cannot sit back and complacently accept that terminally ill patients suffering unbearably should just continue to suffer for the good of society as a whole. We must find a solution to the unbearable suffering of patients whose needs cannot be met by palliative care.

Taking a different kind of view, his fellow peer, the fertility expert Lord Winston, argued:

> My mother is 93. She slips in and out of a pre-dementia situation. During a lucid period some months ago, she said to me, 'I have finally reached the end.' She then became very confused and aggressive and didn't know where she was. Only last week she finds that she is enjoying life again. We cannot predict how people may feel about the future and to take that view is ultimately the most presumptuous thing we can do.

The conflicting views expressed by these members of the House of Lords are mirrored in larger society. The British Medical Association (BMA), the doctors' organisation for the UK, has traditionally been opposed to physician-assisted suicide, arguing that it would worsen doctor–patient relationships (Meikle, 2004). In June 2005, however, it dropped this position, although still rejecting the idea of euthanasia. (While not entirely clear, the distinction between assisted suicide and euthanasia seems to lie in the notion that the former involves doctors *giving patients the means* to kill themselves whereas the latter involves the physician directly administering the fatal dose of a drug (Harding, 2005).) Perhaps the end of the BMA's explicit opposition rests to some extent in its acknowledgement of the direction of social opinion. According to a poll by YouGov for the Dignity in Dying group, 76% of respondents from the general population said they were in favour of assisted suicide provided safeguards were in place (Woodward, 2006). Among doctors themselves, in another poll conducted for the Voluntary Euthanasia Society, 45% thought that helping patients to die when they were suffering unbearably was acceptable. In the same poll, 45% also thought that they had colleagues who had supported assisted suicide, while 27% had been asked for help by patients who wanted to die (Meikle, 2004.)

Q.In the polls above, 76% of general population respondents thought that, with certain conditions, assisted suicide should be legal. The number of doctors who responded in this way was 45%. Assuming polling conditions were the same in each poll, which is unknown, why do you think a lesser number of doctors agreed with assisted suicide?

I began this case study by suggesting that it was one in which many people would clearly see the relevance of values and ethics. Health care professionals, perhaps most likely (but not necessarily always) doctors, may have to face the choice of allowing a fellow human to continue suffering unbearably or supporting a patient's decision to end their life. Thinking about this choice, it almost immediately extends beyond the law, for the legal position is relatively clear: neither doctors nor anyone else can help people end their own lives. (This is the position applying in the UK.) So we begin to enter the territory of values. Should we preserve life at all costs? Are there certain circumstances in which life can properly be said to be worth so little that the best possible course would be for it to be ended? Who should make these kinds of decisions? If it is patients themselves, can we trust their judgements? (An opposing view might be how dare we *not* trust their judgement?) If it is to be doctors, what are our grounds for believing that they are trustworthy enough to decide reasonably between life and death on our behalf? This is especially important given our recent history of shocking exposures of medical neglect, and even deliberate evil done under the cover of medicine -- the most terribly dramatic example of this perhaps being the case of mass-murdering GP Harold Shipman (Smith, 2002, 2003).

Thinking about the questions that I have just posed, my guess is that we would each of us hold different views, and we would hold those different views for separate reasons. We cannot resolve or agree on them simply by considering the law, or technical or other kinds of fact. We possess the views that we do because we hold certain kinds of **beliefs** and **values** – about the nature of life and death, about personal choice, about well-being and suffering, about what it is to be a health care professional. Within this complex of beliefs and values are some that we would probably quite easily want to describe as being related to **ethics**.

But while it is likely that most of us will see the place of values and ethics in considering the case of Dr Irwin, there may be some who still wonder about it, at least in terms of personal relevance: 'What has all this got to do with me? I am a health care professional (a nurse, say) but my job is such that I never have, and am never likely, to enter a situation where a patient is asking me to help them die. And if I did, then I would simply go to a higher authority and tell them about what has happened. They would decide what to do. Even if the question were ever in my hands, it would very quickly be out of them.'

In some ways this sounds like a plausible response to the issue of assisted suicide. It is plausible because I would agree that for many health care professionals, the issue has never been and is never likely to become a reality. Paradoxically, the highly dramatic nature of this case study, which has given it such strong resonance in terms of values and ethics, means that we may be unlikely to encounter it in our practice, or if we do, it will be so fundamental and so overwhelming that in all likelihood our instinctive (and very possibly right) reaction will be to seek help.

> Q: 'There's no need to think about this. It'll never happen to me and even if it did, the responsibility would be someone else's.' What problems do you think there might be with this sort of response to the case of assisted suicide?

It seems to me that there are two difficulties with this kind of response. The first relates to our **individual responsibilities** as health care professionals. If we are conscientious and thoughtful practitioners, would we really be happy about completely abdicating responsibility if we were ever to meet this kind of 'life and death' situation? I would agree that it is quite reasonable for us to seek the help of others. Indeed, we may well have a professional obligation to do so (notwithstanding our legal obligation to act in certain kinds of ways). But to pass it over without thought to someone else seems to be denying our sense of professional integrity in a very important way. Part of being a health care professional is surely taking responsibility for thinking carefully about the kinds of situations the patient or client you have 'professed' to serve is facing (Koehn, 1994). I would want to extend this idea and suggest that we need to think carefully not only about the *actual* situations our patients or clients are in, but also about *potential* circumstances that we might encounter. Part of being a thoughtful health care worker is allowing and developing empathy for our patients and clients, and an imagination for the difficulties they face – even the kinds of highly dramatic difficulties I have discussed.

The second reason relates to what I will call the **public responsibilities** involved in being a health care worker, and especially occupying a professional role. In a highly important sense, dramatic questions of life and death are problems *for us all*, whether or not we are health care professionals. I described earlier the YouGov poll in which a large majority of respondents from the general population gave qualified support for the idea of assisted suicide. I would want to argue that this kind of expression of public opinion is of great importance in shaping the views and decisions of those charged with making public policy and enacting the laws that govern our actions. Even though the Joffe bill was blocked, the politicians concerned would have been keenly aware of public opinion, in much the same way that I have already suggested the BMA probably was when it decided to drop its opposition to assisted suicide. The relationship between public opinion and public policy or legislation is a complex one and mediated by many different factors (Cribb, 2005). However, there is no doubt that one way or another, policy makers and legislators in our liberal-democratic society have to listen to the people, for it is the people who provide them with power. Our position as citizens in a democracy allows us to form opinions on matters of life and death and it would seem to be neglectful of our democratic responsibilities if we did not.

But health care professionals have a particular responsibility to shape and influence public policy in relation to matters of health care, including the kinds of 'life and death' issues I have been discussing. This responsibility stems from the power they possess by virtue of their professional training, and the relatively large degrees of autonomy that society allows them (Ham, 2004). Such power means that the views, beliefs and actions of health care professionals hold particular importance in our society. If we as professionals form particular beliefs and have certain views about the nature of life and death, and about living and dying, they will probably be taken very seriously by our fellow citizens.

For these reasons of both individual and public responsibility, it seems very hard to suggest that health care professionals should take little or no interest in the case of Dr Irwin and Mrs Murphy. The fact that they should be interested lies in both their individual and their public interests as health care professionals. These interests, it is clear, extend beyond the factual and descriptive. They lie in the nature of the beliefs we have and the values we hold. The interests are **ethical** ones.

Case Study: Better Living?

I suggested before that the kind of 'life and death' example provided by the Dr Irwin and Mrs Murphy case was *perhaps* the sort of circumstance in which people most easily consider that ethics has a part to play in deciding what to do or how to think. But if I am to justify my assertion that ethics and values should be of concern to everyone in health care, then I need to show that their consideration is relevant in cases where the dilemma *seems to be* not so acute. Indeed, a key theme I am trying to develop in this book is that values and ethics are relevant to all (or at least very nearly all) aspects of health care. It is the idea of the worth of thinking about values and ethics in 'ordinary' health care (which in fact is 'extraordinary in its ordinariness') that I am mainly intending to try to explore.

Towards the end of 2006, *The Observer* newspaper carried a story with the headline, 'NHS must pay for fat children to get surgery' (Revill, 2006b). The National

Institute for Health and Clinical Excellence (NICE) was recommending that, as a case of last resort, severely overweight teenagers should be offered bariatric surgery ('stomach stapling') as a treatment for their obesity.

> Currently, most patients who might be eligible cannot be given surgery as most primary care trusts, which hold treatment budgets, refuse to pay for the £8000 operation. Between 50 and 200 teenagers a year could get treatment. (Revill, 2006b: 1)

Q: • Do you think the National Health Service (NHS) should pay for obese • children and teenagers to have this kind of expensive treatment?

This headline and story appeared on the first page of the newspaper. It's possible that we might start off by responding to it in at least two different ways. On the one hand, we may think that of course the NHS should be paying for this sort of treatment in cases where everything else has failed. We know that obesity leads to a string of health problems for teenagers, problems that will worsen in adult life. These include type 2 diabetes and psychological problems in adolescence itself, and coronary heart disease (CHD), stroke and cancers in adulthood (NHS Centre for Reviews and Dissemination, 2002). Surely, if we can prevent these kinds of problems by offering surgery when all else has failed, this can only be for the good? After all, even simply on the economic terms that seem to be of most concern to the story-writer, the cost of widespread morbidity and early mortality consequent on unchecked obesity will be much greater than the cost of this treatment.

On the other hand, though, we might wonder exactly why the NHS should be paying for this expensive treatment for teenagers who, we may feel, have only themselves to blame. After all, the reasons for obesity are quite clear, aren't they? Obese children eat too much, especially the 'wrong' kinds of food – high in fat, salt and sugar and with little actual nutritional value (NHS Centre for Reviews and Dissemination, 2002). They spend all their time slumped in front of televisions and computers. If only they would change their own behaviour, we would be rid of the problem; so why should we pay when they don't? My guess is that for most health care professionals, if they respond to the story in either of these two ways, it will most likely be the first. Perhaps above anything else, the vast majority of those working in health care are motivated by a desire to do good, to contribute to efforts aimed at producing more health (leaving aside what that might mean for the moment) and at the alleviation of suffering and disease. They will want to prevent the suffering of these teenagers with very real problems and if bariatric surgery is the method of last resort in doing so, then the cost should be borne by the National Health Service. Health care workers may well be reluctant to enter into the process of 'blaming the victim', which seems to play a prominent part in the second sort of response to the story.

Yet closer thought and analysis reveals a much greater complexity than either of these two kinds of initial response allow. Rising levels of childhood obesity are a major concern to planners and policy makers in the United Kingdom (UK) (Department of Health, 2004), as they are in other developed countries. Research demonstrates that the causes of obesity are not simple to isolate (NHS Centre for Reviews and Dissemination, 2002). Over the last 60 years or so, the way in which lives are lived, at least in the developed world, has changed beyond all recognition. We live and work in very different ways from our grandparents or great-grandparents. With regard to diet and food particularly, when, where, how and even why we eat are different now from the situation in, say, the earlier part of the twentieth century. Many people have a much wider variety of food choices available to them and more money to spend on their groceries bill. But work and other pressures of modern life mean that many of us have less time to shop and cook sensibly. Takeaway and so-called junk food have become commonplace (Campbell, 2006; Sweney, 2007). Many people no longer sit down in families and eat together. Fashion, and concern for body image, play a big part for a large number of people in determining how, what and why they eat. In the same edition of the newspaper as the headline story I am discussing, Clarissa Farr, Headmistress of St Paul's Girls' School, condemned the fashion industry's 'deplorable' obsession with ultra-thin sizes:

> 'It is grossly irresponsible that this kind of thinking is encouraged as something desirable,' Farr said. ... Society's obsession with thinness [she added] was 'a form of fundamentalism, a form of extremism. ... This is about pressure to conform'. (Asthana, 2006)

And of course such pressure to conform, along with beliefs that you are failing to do so, can lead to individuals having very problematic relationships with food. So we might very reasonably be led to the view that treating obesity as a narrow problem of individual lifestyle, amenable to highly specific medical or surgical treatment (ideas inherent within one or other of the positions we initially reviewed) is not enough. Towards the end of the story, its writer quotes public health expert Dr Geoff Rayner from City University in London:

> 'We are medicalising something that is actually to do with how we live as a society. People become overweight because of their environment – because we take a car rather than walk – because we spend hours in front of the TV and because we are saturated by the junk food industry. If you take a purely medical approach to this, you start to normalise what is a deeply abnormal state.' (Revill, 2006b)

It seems to me that Rayner's quote exemplifies the difficulties involved in tackling the problem of childhood obesity, and why our responses to it are centrally related to questions of values and ethics. If we are concerned about this problem, or involved with it in some way at the level of policy or professional practice, we are likely to be motivated at least in part by a desire to help people towards what we might broadly call 'better living'. We want people to live longer and more fully, free as far as possible from physical and psychological pain. We want these things and hold them as values partly because they seem to match up with our conceptions of what is meant by 'good human living'.

But while such broad values may be widely shared (and we might be very suspicious of someone who *doesn't* hold them), their exact nature, along with how we go about achieving them, is much more subject to debate. In this case, is 'better living' not being obese? Or is it not being worried by a society that places a premium on certain ways of appearing and behaving? Is our own 'better living' something that we as individuals are essentially responsible for? Or is it something that we share as a responsibility with all the other members of our highly complicated society? Different answers to these questions will lead us towards separate understandings of the nature of the value of 'better living'. For example, if I think that 'better living' involves me doing my best to stay in good physical shape, I will understand it primarily as a value related to **individual responsibility**. If, on the other hand, I understand it as being dependent on collective pressure and effort, I will conceive it as a value that is **socially mediated**.

> Q.• Do you think the value of 'better living' is down to the responsibility of
>   • the individual? Or does society hold a responsibility for the value of
> 'better living' of its members? Or is the responsibility shared in some way?

How I understand the nature of the value of 'better living', and where responsibility for it lies, will lead me to beliefs about what I should do or what attempts I should support to bring about more of the value. If I think of it as a value connected to individual responsibility, I might well support efforts strongly to persuade people towards lives filled with more nutritional food and greater levels of exercise. If I consider it a value that is largely socially mediated, then my concern will be for work that aims to alter social structures that influence (positively or negatively) the value and its production or diminution. For example, I might consider it a good thing to ban advertising of 'junk food', especially to vulnerable consumers such as young people (Campbell, 2006). These issues of what to do to produce more of a desired value are, as I will discuss in Chapter 4, issues of ethics.

So from discussion about a case that perhaps superficially appeared to be fairly clear-cut, we have begun to uncover a range of potential values and a variety of ethical issues. These are likely to frame and influence our actions in the area of teenage obesity, or our decisions about which actions to support. Moreover, I want to continue with my claim, made earlier in relation to the example of Dr Irwin and Mrs Murphy, that the actions and support of *health care professionals* have special ethical importance, simply because of their being professionals. And while I began this particular example with the idea that it appeared to represent a case and a dilemma that was less 'acute' than the 'life and death' situation Mrs Murphy and Dr Irwin found themselves in, this certainly doesn't mean that it's any less important. For what could be more essential to a health care professional than thinking about ways to encourage 'better living', and about the debates over values and ethics that are intimately connected to its promotion?

Case Study: Better Lives?

Joe is 11 years old, autistic and severely developmentally delayed. He lives with his parents in Hertfordshire. His latest obsession is to drive with his father in the family car, listening to cassettes of Albinoni, Vivaldi, the Jam and Abba:

> Joe's obsessions possess him utterly. When I tell him we'll take another drive at five o'clock (five hours away), he pulls up a chair in front of the kitchen clock, sits down to stare at the passing minutes and waits, and points, and asks constantly for reassurance that the moment will come. ... Given the alternatives that day, there is no realisable purpose or pleasure capable of supplanting the car, or even interrupting his long – sometimes very long – anticipation of its meandering bliss. By comparison, Jeremy Clarkson is an Amish. (Blastland, 2006: 33)

Michael Blastland is Joe's father. In an essay published in the *New Statesman* magazine in April 2006, he reflects on the nature of Joe's life, and the extent to which it squares up with an understanding of what it is to be human, and to live a human life:

> You can run through the philosopher's common measures of what it means to be one of us and find either that Joe fails them outright, or that his inclusion is in doubt. Humanity has deep structured language, it is said; Joe does not. Human beings have complex morality; Joe demonstrates time and again, sometimes brutally, a frail grasp of moral norms and instincts, mostly because he lacks an adequate appreciation of how his behaviour affects others. We have rich self-consciousness; Joe has little if any concern for how others see him and scant reflection, I suspect, on his own thoughts. It is also said that people are, above all, social creatures whose relationships are uniquely subtle and sophisticated. Joe, according to the dominant theories of autism, might be unaware that other people have any kind of mental life, might be blind to the existence of others' minds, and thus incapable of understanding their behaviour or making sense of social situations. (Blastland, 2006: 33)

Thinking About...

Joe has little or no sense of self, or of relationships with others. Consider the effect this might have on our understanding of him as a fellow human being.

Does this mean that Joe can't be said to be human? This question is at the centre of the debate that Michael Blastland has with himself, both in this essay and in a book on which the essay is based (Blastland, 2007). As Joe's father, Blastland's deliberations are framed completely by the love that he has for his son. Indeed, it is this love, and the closeness to Joe it gives him, that provides him with at least part of the answer to the question. Joe is loved and in the love between father and son, meaning for the life emerges. Love gives the life potential. More widely, we all recognise this potential (or at least we all ought to, argues Blastland): 'We define Joe not only by what he can understand or could have hoped for, but what you and I can understand or could have hoped for.' (Blastland, 2006: 35).

This might all sound a bit vague and mystical, but the reality is that a life like Joe's challenges us to ask important questions. In the first place, we need to ask whether we agree with what Michael Blastland seems to be asserting; does the meaning of Joe's life depend on the meaning given it by others? Is it right (or even possible) to talk about life's meaning being wholly ascribed not by the individual whose life it is, but by other people? It is certainly true that *some* of life's meaning is given to me not by myself but by others and how they see me (as kind or as funny, for example), the relationships I have with them, and so on. But I also gather meaning through what might be called my 'inner life' of thoughts and feelings and emotions. What if I was suddenly stripped of all those things? At the very least, I would want to say that if this happened to me, my life would be much less rich. I might even want to say that this wasn't my life at all. The truth is probably that the meaning of my life depends on a mix of the meaning I give to it and that which others ascribe to it. So what if, as in Joe's case, the former is absent?

This leads us to the second question. If I can imagine that for me the absence of my own 'inner life' would make my life much less rich at the very least, it's possible that others might also take this view. So does this mean that such a life (the kind of life Joe has) is *less* valuable than other lives because the inner dimension is missing? One possible way of responding to this question is with a further one; if we had the choice, would we want more or less of the kinds of lives that Joe represents to be created? Many might take the view that we should do what we can to avoid the creation of lives that, as they see it, would be blighted by disability or dysfunction. And it would certainly seem perverse to suggest that we actually wanted *more* severely autistic babies to be born into the world. If this seems like entry into potentially dangerous territory, that is because it is. There is danger for two reasons. First, if we say that we have no desire to see more severe autism in the world, it is not that much of a further step to suggesting that we actually want *less*. This certainly implies a wish or a willingness to alter the patterns of lives being born. And this wish or willingness is something that, at least in theory, could be enacted. It appears to be the case, from research, that autism has a basis in genetics (Wheelwright and Baron-Cohen, 2001). If this is so, then we could conceive of this genetic basis being altered or modified through the immense capabilities we have to hand as a result of advances in reproductive and genetic technology (Cohen, 2006). Wanting (and possibly having the power) to create less of certain kinds of lives (and by implication more of other kinds) should stop and make us think about the desirability of these sorts of wishes and projects.

This leads us to the second reason why the territory is dangerous. If we believe that there might be worth in trying to create less of certain kinds of lives, where do we draw the line? We know that in more or less complex ways, changes in the sequence of genes cause a range of diseases and disabilities, including cystic fibrosis, epilepsy, Down syndrome and Huntington's disease (Cohen, 2006). Should we aim to eliminate this whole range of disorders with genetic components? Should we be aiming for the creation of non-disordered, 'normal' human beings? But what do we mean by 'normal'? Isn't part of being human having to cope with a world in which disability and disease is present? Isn't it a human duty to love and care for those who are born to us, even if (as in Michael Blastland's case), that new person is profoundly disabled?

We do not have to search very far into the past to recognise that history is filled with examples of people and nations that believed 'normality' was constituted by a certain kind of being. For the Nazi regime, being Jewish (or homosexual, or gypsy) was not normal and so Europe saw the extermination of six million people as these 'abnormalities' were dealt with (Burleigh, 2001). It is this really quite recent past that is part of what lies at the heart of concerns about the new genetics and the potential it has for allowing us to create so-called designer babies (Glover, 2006).

If talk of Nazi eugenics and 'designer babies' seems far from the case of Joe and his obsession with car rides, there is a need to be reminded of how easily we got to this position. If Joe's life has meaning only because it means something to others, and this is not the case with the majority of people, then we could argue that his life is *different* from others. If it is different, we could potentially take the view that it holds less **value**. Holding less value, we might assert that we should try to avoid such lives being created. But if we agree with this assertion, we might also agree that we should do our best to avoid the creation of a whole range of lives that are different, that don't conform to our conceptions of 'normality'.

Thinking About...

On page 2, I asked whether you agreed (or otherwise) with my claims that everyone involved in health care should have a concern with values and ethics, and that unless this is present we are not properly engaged in health care at all. Reflect on whether your consideration of these three case studies has altered your initial position in any way.

Conclusion: The Challenge of Values and Ethics

The case of Joe should make us do very much more than just worry about the implications of 'high-tech' genetic engineering projects. It should make us reflect, as health care students or workers, about the value we place on certain kinds of lives. This also applies to the other two case studies within the chapter, concerning assisted suicide and the end of life, and childhood obesity. In all of the cases, individuals (or groups or populations) confront us with strong values related to their lives, their behaviour and their circumstances. Dr Irwin and Mrs Murphy are asking us to see the value of physical life as diminished through painful suffering. Actors in the case of childhood and teenage obesity are demanding that we see lives affected by the problem as both valuable and vulnerable. They also pose the question of who has responsibility for seeking 'better living' for those faced with the consequences of obesity. Joe's father is asking that we share his conception that a life without seeming regard for others is valuable because we make it so.

The people in these case studies are not simply presenting us with their own values. I want to argue that they are also requiring us (either explicitly or implicitly) to be clear about our own values. They want to know whether we share their values, or whether our own are different and, if so, how and why. In turn, they want to know what action we will take to reinforce their values, or to promote our own (or those of the policy makers and managers controlling our work). They want to know these things for a very simple reason. It is this:

If health care is about creating better lives (or at least making the conditions of living and dying more tolerable), then there is a need to know what motivates us in our work, and why we take the decisions and act in the ways that we do.

The case studies that I've presented here could be replicated and extended many times over, but they all lead us towards a pressing requirement to respond to this demand. By virtue of what health care is, and what it aims to do, this demand faces us in every health care-related situation. If we are serious about our work, and respectful of the patients or clients with whom we are involved, we have a duty to respond. It would be showing disrespect not to try to do so. This is the basis for my assertion that everyone involved in health care should have a fundamental concern with issues of values and ethics. **We need to examine the values that underpin our actions, and the ethics of those actions themselves, because they are responses to the task of creating better (or more tolerable) lives – and these lives are valued, one way or another, by those whose lives they are.** The task now is to clarify how this challenge can be met.

Chapter Summary

In this chapter, I have:

- Used a number of case studies to exemplify the view that questions of values and ethics permeate all aspects of health care, from prevention to acute treatment;
- Developed and defended the view that, as a consequence, values and ethics are central to the study and practice of health care;
- Encouraged you to think about the essential importance of exploring your own values and ethical positions as a fundamental response to the 'valuable lives' of the patients or clients with whom you actually or will potentially work.

Further Reading

Dworkin, R (1995). *Life's Dominion: An Argument about Abortion and Euthanasia*. London: HarperCollins. This is a beautifully written and argued book setting out positions in relation to these issues of 'life and death' ethics.

Seedhouse, D (1998). *Ethics: The Heart of Health Care* (Second Edition). Chichester: Wiley. By way of contrast, much of Seedhouse's focus in this book is on the 'everyday' ethics of health care.

2

VALUES, HEALTH AND HEALTH CARE

Learning Outcomes

By the end of this chapter, you should be able to:

○ Identify, describe and discuss what is meant in talking about 'values';
○ Discuss, especially as health care professionals (or professionals-in-training), how values are acquired;
○ Describe and discuss different ways in which it is possible to understand, and talk about, the value of health;
○ Understand the nature of the connection between values, on the one hand, and ethics, on the other, with particular reference to the health care context.

Introduction

I argued in Chapter 1 that questions of values and ethics were central to each of the three case studies I spent time thinking about. These case studies, I also argued, were only representative of much more extensive values-related debates that are taking place all the time in relation to almost every health care situation we might encounter or be involved with. So values are fundamental to, and embedded in, the whole practice of health care.

But if we are serious about any exploration of values in health care, we need first of all to understand what values actually *are*. Where do they come from? Why do we hold the values that we do? Why do others possess values that are different from our own? These are some of the questions that I will spend part of this chapter trying to address. In the light of these discussions about the nature of values, I want to think about how we might understand **the value of health** *itself*. Can we expect unified understanding? If not, what different perceptions might exist and why exactly is the value disputed and contested? Thinking about these questions leads us back into the territory of health care, with all its ambiguities and difficulties. Finally, I want to think a little about the relationship between **values,** on the one hand, and **ethics,** on the other. Are they connected and, if so, how? Is the link uncomplicated or does it create problems for further understanding and exploration? I want to argue that questions related to the connection between values and ethics pose major difficulties for understanding the nature and purpose of ethics itself. The debates in this chapter provide a springboard for future arguments through the book about values and ethics in the context of health care.

What are Values?

The simple and obvious answer to this question is that they are those things we value, or are able to find value in. The *Oxford Dictionary* talks about values as:

> The amount of money or other commodity or service etc. considered to be equivalent to something else for which a thing can be exchanged ... Desirability, usefulness, importance ... The ability of a thing to serve a purpose or cause an effect. (Oxford University Press, 1983: 748).

Like many apparently straightforward definitions, though, these ones prompt us to more questions than they provide answers. If something is desirable, is that the same as it being useful or important? Is it possible for something to be one of these things, but not the others? This seems highly likely. The train that I catch home from work in the evening is useful and important to me as it gets me back to my house (and so for myself it has value), but I'd be reluctant to say that, in itself, it was *desirable*. (Perhaps I might if I was a train enthusiast. But if there is any desirability for me in this example, it lies in what the train *does* – it gets me back home, where I want or desire to be – rather than what it *is* – a particular locomotive class, or a particular configuration of coaches, say.)

This rather simplistic example points up some important things. First, it seems to suggest that there may be **different kinds of values**. We may value something because of its desirability or its importance or its usefulness, but if something is valuable to me, say, it certainly doesn't have to be all of those things (although I would argue that it has to be at least one of them to possess value). Second, it points to the idea that different people are likely to value different things, and even if they hold the same thing as valuable, they may value that thing in different ways. To emphasise this idea further, take the final component of the definition above – something possessing value because it serves a purpose or causes an effect. To me, the ability to read is a value. It is a value because it gives me great pleasure, allows me to escape into alternative worlds, and so on. These are the effects that reading has on me, and this is more often than not my purpose in sitting down to read. For somebody else, the value of the ability to read lies solely in its allowing them to make sense of the world, to follow instructions, to navigate their way through public transport systems, and so on. For this other person, that value can be described (in terms of purpose and effect) simply in those ways. It can be described like that for me as well. (After all, where would I be if I couldn't read the instruction manual for my washing machine or work out where I was going on the Tube?) But I would need to 'add in' the extra bits of description, such as pleasure and so on, in forming my own account of the value of the ability to read.

Much philosophical work has gone into trying to understand the nature of values. The moral and legal philosopher Ronald Dworkin has developed a useful account of values and their nature. He argues (Dworkin, 1995) that there are three kinds of values:

- Subjective values;
- Instrumental values;
- Intrinsic values.

Subjective values are those that relate to preference or 'liking' (Downie et al., 1996). A value is **instrumental** if the thing that I value has usefulness for me. Something holds **intrinsic value** if we cannot reduce that value to considerations of preference or of utility. We might regard this kind of value as applying to things that are so essential to being human that talk of liking or usefulness of the value seems absurd; we just know this thing, whatever it might be, has fundamental (intrinsic) value. Something might have *only* subjective or instrumental or intrinsic value, or it might possess a combination of these.

Perhaps examples might help to develop our understanding of Dworkin's classification. I have deliberately chosen 'non-health' examples for the time being in order to allow us to focus on the nature of valuing itself before I move on to consider the shape of values that might be related to health and health care. Let's go back to the train I catch to and from work – my daily commute. Imagine I'm returning home quite late one evening after spending the day meeting and teaching students. I'm tired but in good spirits. As I cross the station concourse, I catch sight of a stall that sells sweets and drinks. Suddenly I think that I fancy a chocolate bar. I don't need one – I'm not at all hungry – it would just be nice to have. That chocolate bar would have **subjective value** for me. I just happen, at that moment, to have a liking for the taste of chocolate and a preference for this kind of snack over, say, a bag of crisps, or something else that would be far, far better for me!

I buy the chocolate bar and head for the train. I want to suggest, as I implied before I introduced Dworkin's classifications, that the train possesses **instrumental value**. It has usefulness or utility for me in that it takes me (usually with not that much fuss) from home to work and back again. Of course it might also have subjective value; I greatly prefer travelling by this train to driving through congested city streets to reach my workplace, but if I were asked to think about the train's value to me I would probably do so in instrumental terms.

Imagine now that it is some time later and I finally arrive home. The curtains are drawn at the windows of my house and I can see the dim glow of lamps through them. I open the front door and there is a shout of welcome. It's warm inside. One of the family makes me a cup of tea and I sit down in a comfortable chair to drink it. All of the things that I've mentioned – the warmth, the welcome, the cup of tea, the comfortable chair – have instrumental and subjective value to me. But they also embody the idea of *home*, and I want to suggest that the value of home (and the things it represents) extends beyond subjectivity or instrumentality. Its value is arguably **intrinsic**. The nature of humanity and being human is such that 'home' possesses fundamental value. It provides warmth, shelter, companionship, love, and so on. Of course the value of home (and associated values) might also be thought of as instrumental. For example, the fact that I possess them helps me to get on with my life and work in ways that I might not be able to do if I was in different circumstances. However, I can't see them wholly in these terms and others might be shocked if I tried to do so. What if I said that my home and family were valuable to me only in so far as they helped me to get on with my own life? At best, I would be thought cold and calculating. The truth seems to be that the value of 'home', and many of the values associated with it, might not be reducible to ideas of preference or utility.

> Q: What are the things you value in your own life? Construct a list, trying to classify the things on your list according to whether you think their value is subjective, instrumental or intrinsic (or a combination of more than one of these things). If you have any difficulties in coming up with your classifications, ask yourself why this might be the case.

The problem of intrinsic value

One of the difficulties that might have emerged in the process of thinking about values and what is valuable in your own life may have been that of trying to get to the heart of what might have **intrinsic value**. It's possible that you were easily able to identify things that have subjective and instrumental value for you, but that it was much harder to alight on things that might be regarded as intrinsically valuable. More particularly, is it right to suggest that there are values whose worth lies mainly or wholly in their intrinsic nature? For example, it's possible that one of the things you might have come up with in your 'values list' is the value of the education that you might be currently acquiring, or have acquired in the past. But is it right to talk about 'the value of education' as valuable in itself? Surely, we value education because of what it does for us; it makes us more employable, gives us skills to cope with life, perhaps for some is enjoyable (and so also has a subjective, 'liking' or aesthetic value). Going back to the example that I provided earlier of some of my own values, I argued that the idea and reality of 'home' had intrinsic value for me. But is this really the case? Can I actually think of 'home' in any other way than the subjective and instrumental value that it provides for me (warmth, companionship, shelter, all of which I enjoy and need in order to get on with life)?

Philosophers themselves have had long struggles with the idea of intrinsic value, trying to tease out what it actually means (Audi, 2004; Baird-Callicott, 2005; Williams, 2002). They have tried to suggest that intrinsic values are those which can be recognised as such from an impersonal or general point of view (Williams, 2002). For example, 'truth' has value for me because of its instrumentality. It is important for me that the person waiting at the bus stop is telling the truth about the time of the next bus, otherwise I will miss it. Equally, it is important that I tell the truth to the person who comes up to the stop and asks me about the times. If I have previously lied to her, the next time I'm in a fix about bus schedules, I might ask the very same person and on the basis of her past experience, she may well go ahead and lie back to me. But the value of truth telling lies beyond its personal use to me. I can see the value of telling the truth in a whole range of situations that don't concern me at all. Thus 'truth' assumes a general or impersonal value. We might call this argument for the nature of intrinsic values the **general recognition** argument.

Again, and somewhat in contrast, other philosophers have tried to frame intrinsic values as those things in our lives that make living them worthwhile (Audi, 2004). Continuing with the 'truth' example, if I live a life in which the value of truth plays an essential part (I believe it is fundamental that I do my best to tell the truth in all situations, and so on), this will contribute to the nature of my life as worthwhile. On the other hand, if I imagine living a life in which truth plays no part at all, where my existence is riddled with lies and deceit and the effects of these things, then for me this won't constitute a worthwhile life at all. This is because of the kind of value that 'truth' is. By this account, the worth of intrinsic values lies in our *experience* of them as formulators of 'lives that are worth living' (Audi, 2004: 123). We could call this argument for the nature of intrinsic values the **experience of worthwhile living** argument.

The contrast between the two arguments for the nature of intrinsic values should now be clear. The 'general recognition' argument does not depend on our necessarily having experience in our own lives of the value suggested as intrinsic; we can impersonally recognise its intrinsic worth for the peace and progress of humanity. The 'experience of worthwhile living' argument, on the other hand, obviously does depend on us having (if only by proxy) a sense of the experience of living 'the worthwhile life' through these values (or what it would be like if these values were absent from our lives).

> Q: Can you think of any difficulties with these two arguments for the nature of intrinsic values – on the one hand, that they are those which require 'general recognition' and, on the other, that they are those we need to possess in order to lead 'worthwhile lives'?

It seems to me that the problem with both arguments is that neither of them makes it very clear what might actually count as an intrinsic value. Sticking with the 'truth' example, what is it about truth that makes us suggest that it should hold general recognition as an intrinsic value? There are occasions when truth actually doesn't have value. Imagine that I know the person asking me about bus times is a suspect in a crime (I recognise her face from photographs on posters). Surely, rather than helping her to move with ease, I should be offering false information so that I have time to go and call the police and she can then be arrested? Equally, it seems difficult to suggest that there is just one set of values connected to the experience of living 'the worthwhile life'. We would probably more reasonably believe there is a range of values that might or might not contribute to the experience of worthwhile living, depending on the particular context of the life concerned (and thus that might be regarded as intrinsic).

One way out of these problems might be to argue that something has intrinsic value when all other kinds of value (for example, instrumental) have been stripped away from it (Baird-Callicott, 2005). If we agree with this, then both the 'general recognition' and 'the experience of worthwhile living' arguments for the nature of intrinsic values become less difficult. What matters is not so much whether we are able to generally recognise a value as intrinsic; or have direct experience of the nature of the value that suggests to us it is intrinsic. Rather, what counts is whether our analysis of any value we choose to examine will result in us being able to see it as disconnected from any consideration of usefulness, preference, and so on.

Thinking About...

Take one of the things from the list you constructed earlier of what is of value in your own life. Thinking as carefully as possible, try to disentangle usefulness, preference, liking, and so on from this value so that it stands independently of these things and therefore might possess *intrinsic* value.

The Acquisition of Values

It is possible, though, that even applying this level of close thought to a value or values will not yield the conclusion that the value concerned is intrinsic. Or at least, we can't deny that such a conclusion might be disputed. I might have satisfied myself that 'family', say, has intrinsic value. However, somebody could come along and assert that if I *really* thought about it, I would recognise that I always have to connect the value of 'family' back to thoughts of its use to me or to wider society, my enjoyment of the comfort it brings, and so on. The point is that I could pare down something to what I believe is its ultimate intrinsic value, but the result of my exercise might well be challenged.

Reaching the position that it is hard (if not impossible) to identify a definitive set of intrinsic values – values that are so important we cannot reduce them to questions of preference or usefulness – is by no means a dispiriting one. What it serves to emphasise is that the form and nature of values can always be disputed. This is especially important in relation to health and health care, where experience tells us that there is much disagreement about what is important, and about what should be done and how we should do it. If we recognise such disagreement as emerging from differences in values, then its strength and its long-lasting nature will become much more explicable because we have seen how slippery and difficult values and their analysis can be. In order to begin to understand and untangle the nature of such disagreement (although not necessarily to resolve the disagreement itself) an important thing to do now is to try to work out **how and why values are acquired.**

Q: • What do you think are the sources of the values that you hold?

Your answers here are likely to have produced a *range* of possible sources of your values. These might have included places of education (school, college, university) or places of informal education, family and friends, local community, media, religious groups, political parties, professional mentors or peers, and so on. Each of these (and other sources that you might have thought about) is likely to be powerful in shaping what we actually value (Halstead and Reiss, 2003).

Generally speaking, Western societies are founded and work on a framework of what we might call **liberal values.** While liberalism itself is hard to define, it is widely accepted as involving a set of values that place individuals and their freedom at the centre of debate and decision-making about what is important and what should be done. So a 'list' of liberal values would probably include things like personal autonomy, openness, equality of opportunity, democracy, and so on (Halstead and Reiss, 2003). However, there is a need to recognise that while these kinds of values are widely accepted and viewed as crucial for the proper functioning of our society, they are not *universally* agreed upon. Even if we agree that the kinds of values I've just listed are important, we might well dispute the exact nature of that value. For example, I might agree with the value of democracy, but would I be happy about a political party with very extreme views (to do with 'race', say) being allowed to participate, at least without some constraint, in the democratic process? Even within our liberal society, values associated with liberalism might be widely accepted, but not necessarily by everybody. Nor is there likely to be uniform agreement on their exact nature.

At least part of the reason for this lies in the fact that while we might all be members of a liberal society, precisely how we acquire particular values – who or what mediates or transmits them to us – will vary from person to person. Two strong sources of values identified by Halstead and Reiss (2003) are religion (of whatever particular kind) and the family. To demonstrate the significance of these sources and how they can profoundly shape the values of those influenced by them, consider this example. Suppose that Bert has been brought up within a strongly evangelical Christian family. His father had very definitely been the head of the family. His mother had never gone out to work and had always deferred in any matter to her husband. The whole family had gone to church every Sunday, and Bert had attended Bible classes and youth groups regularly during the week. The biblical message and biblical values were conveyed strongly at each of these occasions, and enacted at home. Now think about Diane, brought up in a family where religion has no significance at all, and where both her mother and father went out to work, brought home equal amounts of money and took equal part in all family-related decisions.

It is easy to imagine Bert and Diane emerging from their separate experiences of childhood and youth with quite different views about the nature and limits of so-called liberal values, as well as particular values inspired by their own family and religious histories. For example, Bert might believe that there are strict limits to the value of autonomy, so that complete personal licence and freedom can't be allowed in, say, sexual relationships. Sex is only permissible after you have married someone. Diane, on the other hand, might believe that freedom extends to all areas of life, including choices and decisions about when she has sex, and with whom she has it.

Of course, somebody could argue that this is a rather simplistic view of the outcome of childhood experiences of religious and family values. We could imagine that either Bert or Diane (or both), as adults with the capacity to value as they wish and enact their own lives, might adopt contrary values to the ones anticipated by their development. At the very least, they might pursue and agree with a set of 'middle of the road' values that could turn out to have much in common with liberalism in the general sense I described before.

I certainly don't want to deny the possibility (very often a reality) of people shaping and deciding their values for themselves. On the other hand, there is a need to recognise the complex interplay between what we might call individual personality and the culture, institutions and society in which that personality dwells (Tones and Green, 2004). If this is recognised and accepted, then what matters about the Bert and Diane example is not so much what particular values they hold at the moment. What is important is our belief that these have emerged, and have the particular nature that they do, precisely because of the entwining of our individual selves with the family, culture and society within which we have grown up and live.

Values and Health Care Professionals

But there is another dimension to the acquisition of values in the case of those professionally involved in health care, or training for such involvement. It is that the process of professional training *in itself* inculcates, or further strengthens, particular values, or ways in which values are regarded (Duncan, 2007).

One of the things any health care professional has in common with another is that they will both have undergone a lengthy period of training and education before being accredited and allowed to practise independently. This applies to doctors, nurses, pharmacists, physiotherapists, occupational therapists and the whole range of professionals working in health care. Indeed, we can regard this lengthy training as one of the 'traits' of being a professional, along with others such as specialised skills, and a body of specialist knowledge to which the professionals concerned alone have proper access (Hoyle, 1980). This education and training (often undertaken in arduous conditions and at highly formative points of peoples' lives) has broadly two outcomes:

- Professionals learn what to do and how to do it;
- They learn what to **believe** and what to **value** (Duncan, 2007: 25–26).

This second outcome of professional education and training is especially important for our discussion about the nature and acquisition of values, so it requires a little more discussion. When somebody begins a course of professional training and education, to qualify as a nurse, say, they obviously start to study explicit bodies of knowledge – what we might call 'nursing or nursing-related knowledge'. Leaving aside debates about the exact nature of nursing knowledge (and even whether specific nursing knowledge is possible) (Edwards, 2001), we can suggest that nurses need to have the kind of knowledge that will enable them to do their job. Once again, there might be debates about what the job – the purpose or 'ends' of nursing – actually is. But let's assume, from Steven Edwards, that 'plausible candidates' for the ends of nursing include: 'The relief of suffering, promotion of well-being, fostering autonomy' (Edwards, 2001: 9).

To do this job, to achieve these ends, we need certain kinds of knowledge. We need to know how the body works, and how and why it sometimes fails to work (anatomy and physiology). We need to know how and why people function, or find difficulty in functioning, as well as having a clear view of what 'human functioning' is itself (psychology, sociology and philosophy). We also need practical knowledge, that is to say, knowledge enabling us to perform professional actions that help relieve suffering, promote well-being and foster autonomy.

Thinking About....

Consider what are, or might be, the ends of your own profession and the kind of knowledge required to achieve these. (If your profession happens to be nursing, consider your reactions to the account above of possible nursing ends and knowledge.)

In responding carefully to this exercise, you will have started to examine and reflect on the purpose of what you do, and as part of this you will have begun to encounter the beliefs you have as a professional, and the values that you hold. For example, imagine that you regard the end (the purpose) of nursing as the relief of suffering. It will be easy to believe, then, in the importance to nursing of knowledge of morbid anatomy and how to deal with people in morbid states (say, somebody who has difficulty in breathing). Such knowledge will thus also assume a value. So the connection between the two outcomes of professional training and education that I described above becomes clear.

The story, however, does not end there. It is relatively easy to imagine health care professionals (or professionals-in-training) valuing the knowledge they hold and the skills they practise. If they didn't, it would be quite reasonable to ask why they were actually doing the job (or training to do it) in the first place. But the type and nature of values held by health care professionals extend well beyond the relatively narrow valuing of particular kinds of knowledge and skill. They extend into what might be called the values of the profession itself.

Let's continue with the nursing example. If I am a nurse, it would be hard for me to accept the value of knowledge and skill related to the relief of suffering if I didn't believe that such relief (one of the potential ends of the profession) was a value itself. We could add to this list of the potential values of nursing by thinking about some of the other things on Edwards' list of nursing ends, or purposes. If nursing is about promoting well-being, then surely well-being itself must be a value. If it's about fostering autonomy, then autonomy has to be a value. We could add to this list further values such as caring, individual welfare, and so on (Duncan, 2007).

My argument now is that the values on this kind of list are not only central to the profession of nursing, but also key to each member of that profession. The same applies across the range of health care professions. If your profession has well-being as one of its central values, then you are likely to share this value (leaving aside for the moment the very thorny question of what 'well-being' actually *is*). To accept this is partly common sense. (Again, how could it be possible to live the life of a professional and be in constant dispute and disagreement with your profession's values?). But my argument is also rooted in a view of how professional values are actually *acquired*.

Health care professionals learn what to value (as well as how to value it) in two different ways: through what might be called the **'explicit' curriculum**; and through what we might regard as the **'hidden' curriculum** (Cribb and Bignold, 1999). The 'explicit' curriculum, as the term implies, is constituted by what is formally taught in both the academic and the professional components of any period of professional training. The 'hidden' curriculum is what is being conveyed about the profession, what it does, why it exists and individuals' places within it in non-formal or informal ways. The 'hidden' curriculum is conveyed and enacted in conversations about patients and other staff during coffee breaks, or in comments about standards of dress by a ward sister to students working on her ward. It is delivered when an occupational therapist is encouraged to write up her patient notes in a certain way, or when a medical social worker's colleagues eye him a little suspiciously as he leaves the office slightly earlier than he should. It is, in other words, a set of unwritten rules that govern development and behaviour in a profession (Duncan, 2007) and to which the professional or professional-in-training has to conform (at least to some extent) if they want to survive and thrive.

If you were to be asked to about your experience of the 'explicit' and the 'hidden' curricula in your own professional training and development, it is highly possible that you will be able to identify and recall the 'hidden' experience much better than the 'explicit' one. I want to suggest that, in general, our 'socialisation into professional values' (Hoyle, 1980) is much more effectively and powerfully done through the 'hidden' curriculum than through our explicit training and educational experiences. For myself, training as a nurse a number of years ago now, I remember the long night duties sharing the care of a terminally ill patient, say, or the lecture you got from the ward sister for arriving late on a shift, much better than many of the hours of lectures and teaching sessions that we passed through. It was the powerful informal socialisation, the 'hidden' curriculum, that very largely shaped my views on the nature of nursing and the values of the profession.

Of course I do not mean to imply that the formal or 'explicit' curriculum is unimportant. Quite the opposite, in fact, for the thoroughgoing socialisation into a profession and its values that happens to professionals-in-training is actually a result of a powerful interplay between explicit and 'hidden' curricula. We learn what to know and do largely through explicit teaching; and we learn what to believe and how to value what we know and do through the 'hidden' curriculum (Duncan, 2007).

The Values of Health Care

The argument I have constructed for the acquisition of values by health care professionals begins to suggest that these values are powerfully transmitted and become deeply embedded in our lives and work. A number of studies have explored and confirmed this idea (see, for example, Becker et al. (1977) writing about medical students undergoing this process, or Clouder (2003) discussing the development of occupational therapy students).

Q: What values do you think are important in health care, and for those working in the field? Take one of the values that you have identified and try to consider what might be its *exact* nature.

In responding to this question, it is highly likely that a fundamental point of reference as you tried to develop a clearer conception of the particular value you identified would have been your professional experience. Say, for example, that you chose to try to unpack the value of 'caring' (which we might reasonably assume to be an important value within health care). Possibly, at least part of your framing of the value of 'caring' would have involved seeing it as the task of looking after people so they benefit from the expertise that you possess as a professional (or a professional-in-training). It is hard to see how this kind of conception could not have been at least partly formed by the powerful experiences inherent in the process of professional training that I have just been discussing. Equally, if you resist this conception, and instead view that version of the value of 'caring' as controlling and paternalistic, you will still be making strong reference to the value as it has been played out in your experiences and observations on wards and in clinics. We cannot escape from our profession, whatever it is, and the ways that it has moulded our conceptions of values, as both acceptance and tales of resistance show (see, for example, Armstrong (1983) and the story of his challenge as a young doctor to what he characterises as medicine's overarching values of control and surveillance).

All this leads us to a position in which we can see the values of health care as ardently held and also, when disagreement occurs, heavily disputed. Yet despite this, we may well continue to believe (and want to believe) there are some values that are central to the practice of health care, and of core importance, over which genuine dispute would be difficult. What might these be?

Once more, in the same way that we did in thinking about the relationship between purpose, knowledge, beliefs and values in relation to the profession of nursing, we have to return to the **ends of health care** to try to understand what its core values might be. Indeed, Edwards' 'plausible candidates' for the ends of nursing (relieving suffering, promoting well-being and fostering autonomy) (Edwards, 2001: 9) *might be* reasonably put forward as the ends of health care itself. One thing that *can* quite confidently be asserted is that the ends of health care are not health care *itself*. We do not build hospitals, train professionals, develop technology, administer public health systems and so on in order to understand them as ends in themselves. (Given the frequent focus by politicians and policy makers on these instruments of health care, this is not such an obvious point as it might first appear. Governments of all political persuasion are inclined to talk about how many hospitals they have built, say, or about how much they have reduced waiting times, as if these things were in fact the very ends of health care.)

We develop health care, and fund health care systems, broadly so that we can improve health. This very wide conception of the ends of health care leads us back to the kinds of things that Edwards mentions. From these, we can perhaps suggest that the values central to health care include things like autonomy (associated with further values such as free will, respect and consent), caring (also involving compassion and responsibility) and equality (which might also include values of justice and fairness). Certainly, if we accept that the ends of health care are to do with health improvement, then there are some values that we can automatically (or almost automatically) reject. For example, some people would assert that there is value in ethnic identity (which may well be acceptable) and that some such identities have greater value than others (which it is unlikely that we could accept). This latter idea cannot be accepted if we believe that the ends of health care are to do with health improvement, for we know that the discrimination and injustice consequent on the acceptance of such a value will not improve health. (At least, it will not improve health *for all*, which at the moment I am assuming is implicit in our understanding of health improvement as the ends of health care. Any narrowing of this interpretation of health improvement, whatever the reason, is likely to be highly problematic, as I will discuss in Chapter 8.)

So it seems as if there is indeed a set of values that are core to the health care enterprise, accepting that its ends are to do with health improvement. However, this clarity is only fleeting if we move on to the natural next question – what *exactly* do we mean when we talk about 'health improvement'? What is the nature of the value of health, the one value above all others that must surely be central to the health care enterprise?

The literature is rich with philosophical theories of health and its nature as a value (Cribb, 2005; Downie et al., 1996; Nordenfelt, 1993; Scadding, 1988; Seedhouse, 1998, 2001; Wilson, 1975 provide just some examples of this). There is also a very extensive literature that attempts to understand, often through empirical fieldwork, what both professionals and 'lay' people understand by the idea of 'health' (see, for example, Armstrong, 1993; Cox et al., 1987; Herzlich, 1973; Porter, 1995; Williams, 1983). In some senses, this literature can be seen as raising more questions than it offers answers to the extremely vexed question 'What is health?' However, there are some conclusions that can be drawn from these writings, and that can be connected to our own debates about the nature of values, and of values in health care:

- The nature of the value of 'health' is as disputed and disagreed upon as any other health care-related value.
- 'Health' can be understood as a value according to all of the kinds of classifications described by Dworkin, with which I began this chapter. I can see health as a subjective value because if I am healthy – through going to the gym or doing cross-country running, say – I feel better and I *like* having that feeling. I can see it as instrumental in value because it enables me to get on with my life and my daily functioning. And it might appear to have intrinsic value because being healthy (from its etymological roots, being 'whole') seems to tie in with our idea of what it is to be properly human.
- We can understand the nature of 'health' as a value in a range of ways, which can be classified broadly into two. On the one hand, 'health' can be understood as an **objective** phenomenon (health is, say, 'the absence of disease'). On the other hand, what we understand health to be is subject to **interpretation**. This interpretation depends, among other things, on who we are, what kind of society we live in, what gender we possess, and so on. Importantly, there are some who would argue fiercely for health as being no more and no less than an **objective state,** and others who would not waver from asserting that it could be nothing other than **subject to interpretation**. Equally, there are many (and this is a particularly strong feature of lots of 'lay' accounts of health) who see 'health' as a mix of the objective and the interpretative.

As we start on this exploration of the nature of values and ethics in health care, the problem with 'health' taking on this complex and contestable nature – the challenge it offers our discussions – is that it makes the whole enterprise of health care subject to dispute. What should we be doing in health care? How should we be going about it? These questions are central to us but because of the nature of the values of health care, including the value of health itself, they are not at all easy ones for us to try to answer. We can certainly put forward and promote a set of values core to health care, as I have just done. There is good reason to try to do so; after all, we need some kind of compass for our work. But there is no guarantee at all that they will be accepted by everyone, or will remain immune to different interpretation. This is at least partly because of the disputed character of 'health' itself.

Conclusion: Connecting Values and Ethics in Health Care

I have spent some time exploring the nature of values and valuing, starting off with the simple claim that values are, basically put, those things that we find valuable. However, as we start to think about the nature of things that possess value for us, we begin to realise that others might think differently about that value, or even place no value at all on whatever it is that is being considered. So if we assert that we need to engage in health care because it produces things that are valuable, and especially more of the value of 'health' itself, there is a need to be careful on at least two counts:

- Others could disagree about the value of the things actually produced by health care;
- There might well be disagreement about the nature of the value that many see as central to health care and its purposes, that is, the value of 'health' itself.

These difficulties give rise to a clutch of further problems. How do we know what we should be doing in health care? What activities, treatments and interventions *should* we be undertaking? What should we definitely *not* be doing? Why should we be setting limits on treatments and interventions at certain points and not at others? The waters are muddied still further by the fact (demonstrated through empirical evidence) that different kinds of people think in different ways about the nature of the central value of 'health'. For example, 'lay' peoples' views seem to differ in at least some respects from those of health care professionals, although we need to take care because this generalisation does not account for the complexities within separate 'lay' accounts. Look back to the three cases that we thought about in Chapter 1 – Dr Irwin and Mrs Murphy, childhood obesity, and Joe, the severely autistic young boy. It is now clearer that how we think about each case (and therefore what we believe ought to be done about it) is related to values that are, or are likely to be, heavily disputed.

This is the point where it is possible to begin connecting our discussion about values together with ethics. A simple view of the nature of ethics is that it is: 'Enquiry into how [we] ought to act in general' (Lacey, 1976: 60). Ethics is also often understood as enquiry attempting to determine what is valuable, and why it should be regarded as such. This latter purpose of ethics has a clear relevance to our discussions about values, and in particular the disputed values of health care. But so does the former, and there is a need to emphasise the connection between the two purposes to help strengthen our understanding of the links between values and ethics in health care.

In my view, the connection between these two separate purposes of ethics lies in the idea that if we have conceptions of what is valuable, we will want to try to produce more of that value and so we need to know how we ought to act in order to ensure that production. Equally, we will want to avoid or limit the possibilities of producing things that will conflict with what we see as valuable. But this enterprise again poses difficulties:

- How do we determine what is valuable?
- What do we do to increase 'the valuable' (whatever it is)?

These difficulties are demonstrated by thinking again about just one of the cases in Chapter 1. Somebody might argue that Mrs Murphy was in such pain, in a place so remote from our ordinary understanding of what it is to be human, that she no longer put any value on her own life and its continuation and that we should agree her life had become without value. Thus Dr Irwin was right in helping her to kill herself. However, somebody else could argue that always, in every circumstance, human life has value simply because it is human and therefore the killing was wrong.

This brief reflection on the case starts to emphasise the important connection between the two purposes of ethics: determining what is valuable and working out what to do to create more of the valuable. It also begins to pose another set of questions, this time more especially to do with action. If we want to produce more of 'the valuable' (whatever this is), do we pay particular attention to the likely **consequences** of our action? Or does the valuable lie in performing action that we believe to be right **regardless of the consequences**? What kind of action is this likely to be? How will we know when, where and how to perform 'right action'? These are just some of the questions that have preoccupied ethicists through the ages and into our own time. Discussing them in the context of health care is one of the major themes of much of the rest of this book. But before I embark on that task, it is important to think about how and why ethics became important to health care; and how and why health care became important to ethics. Considering history is one of the ways in which we can try to make the present more understandable.

Chapter Summary

In this chapter, I have:

- Described and discussed different kinds of values;
- Discussed how we might acquire, especially as health care professionals or professionals-in-training, the values that we have;
- Reflected on the nature of 'health' as one of the values central to health care;
- Discussed the fundamental connection between values and ethics.

Further Reading

Downie, RS, C Tannahill and A Tannahill (1996). *Health Promotion: Models and Values* (Second Edition). Oxford: Oxford University Press. This is a detailed discussion of the nature of values and how they might impact on public health and health promotion activity in health care.

Halstead, JM and MJ Reiss (2003). *Values in Sex Education: From Principles to Practice*. London: Routledge Falmer. The focus of this book is on the nature of sex education (especially in schools) as a values-laden enterprise. However, it also contains much useful general discussion about the nature of values and how they are acquired.

3

VALUES AND ETHICS IN HEALTH CARE: HISTORICAL PERSPECTIVES

Learning Outcomes

By the end of this chapter, you should be able to:

○ Describe and discuss, in historical terms, key aspects of the relationship between values, ethics and health care;
○ Identify, describe and discuss in particular the reasons for the emergence of the field of bioethics in the mid- to late twentieth century;
○ Describe and discuss the impact of the recent history of doubt and mistrust in the relationship between health care and society on yourself as a health care professional and on the profession to which you belong.

Introduction

Philosophers (including ethicists) are generally quite good at giving the impression that they are the first people ever to have been able to properly reason about the matters they are considering. They might even imply, in what they write and what they say, that their ideas are brand new, never before aired in any lecture hall or read about in any book or journal. My purpose in this chapter is partly to argue that this is not the case; that philosophers are participants in a long tradition that is intimately woven with the social times they inhabited, or are living in now, alongside their (non-philosophical) fellows. The philosopher, I want to argue, is not a remote figure in an isolated ivory tower but somebody who (like the rest of us) is engaged in the hurly-burly of life. Involvement in philosophy (reading, writing, thinking and arguing) just happens to be their response to the messy confusion of our world.

The argument that philosophers are intimately connected with their social times is by no means a new one. The twentieth-century British philosopher Bertrand Russell wrote an entire book in which he traced the history of Western philosophy 'and its connection with political and social circumstance from the earliest times to the present day'. He prefaced the book with a remark:

> Philosophers are both effects and causes; effects of their social circumstances and of the politics and institutions of their time; causes (if they are fortunate) of beliefs which mould politics and institutions of later ages. (Russell, 1979: 7)

Russell is certainly suggesting that some (lucky) philosophers, perhaps by virtue of the novelty or the force of their ideas, have influence on subsequent times. But the important point to note is that the influence, where it exists, is reciprocal. Philosophers and philosophy can change – and sometimes have changed – the world, but the world needs to be ready to be changed. The ideas of Karl Marx, for example, which gave rise to socialist movements that swept nations and really did alter the course of history, emerged in part from his observations of what he saw as the brutality of the English Industrial Revolution. And it was brutalised societies that were ready to accept his ideas and take action against those who controlled them.

The obvious centre of our attention for this argument about philosophy as absolutely bound up in its historical times is the field of health care. Philosophers concerned to explore the nature and value of health and health care, what we should be doing in our field of work and interest and how we should be doing it, are as enmeshed in their times as anybody else. As I will show, philosophical-ethical interests, concerns and direction in relation to health and health care have changed, but these changes are as a result of a complex interplay between thinkers and their society. More often than not, the interplay is heavily in favour of society, with philosophers being led by their times rather than the other way around. This is especially the case in the recent history of the involvement of ethics with medicine and health care; the history of what is often called **bioethics**.

Equally, I argue in the final part of this chapter that you, as a health care worker, cannot escape either the influence of ethics on your work or of the society that has made thinking about ethics such an imperative for those involved in health care. This in turn leads to the idea that 'ethical thinking' is an important element of your occupational or professional persona. A lot of the rest of this book is about developing perspectives and means by which you can reach towards the end of becoming an 'ethical thinker' in the messy and complex world of health care.

Before I move forward, it's necessary to say something about terminology. I will talk about **philosophers** when I want to distinguish them from **moral philosophers** or **ethicists** – people who have a particular interest in moral or ethical thinking. (Philosophy in general also involves other branches apart from ethics, including epistemology (the study of the foundations of knowledge) and metaphysics (the study of being and existence).) I will sometimes talk about **ethics** and sometimes about **moral philosophy**, using the terms interchangeably. While some would disagree with this interchangeable use, it helps make life simpler! In the same way, I will sometimes talk about **moral philosophers** and sometimes about **ethicists**. When I reach the point where the relatively recent project of what is often called **bioethics** begins, I will sometimes use this term, or alternatively **medical ethics** or **health care ethics**. The people involved in this I will generally call **bioethicists**.

Historical Perspectives: The Long View

Philosophy's interest in health and health care is not new. It is possible to trace it back to the earliest Western philosophical writings – the work of the Ancient Greeks. Ancient Greece was not only the birthplace of rational enquiry into the nature of illness and health, but also the time and place that shaped medical ethics and practice even down to our own age. The Hippocratic oath (from the Greek thinker Hippocrates) is still today regarded as central to the ethical purpose of the profession of medicine (Turner, 2003). I want to suggest that there are three separate strands (or what we might call 'narratives') within this long history:

- The history of philosophers trying to understand what 'health' actually *is*;
- The history of how 'health' has been seen, at different times and in different places, as a concept that has particular ethical importance attached to it (that is to say, its history as a value and its relationship to other social values);
- The history of ethics in health care (or rather, perhaps, the history of ethics in medicine, because for a large part of history, health care has – at least in 'official' accounts – largely been *understood as* medicine).

Of course, each of these strands is strongly connected to the others. For example, we might trace, as David Armstrong (2003) does, a change in the way illness was perceived in the late eighteenth century. It altered from being seen as connected with bodily humours (fluids) to its being associated with specific pathological lesions. This re-modelling of 'illness', we could argue, led to a re-modelling of 'health'. Health began to be seen as the absence of pathogens; the absence, in other words, of illness and what had specifically caused illness. So the *value* of 'health', from about that time, might have been seen as resting around disease absence. Moral worth lay in avoiding disease and the pathogens that caused it. Diseases such as tuberculosis, and its causative pathogen the tubercle bacillus, took on a moral significance, as did being TB-free (Tomes, 1997). In turn, this view of the nature and value of health itself (the absence of disease) dictated the purpose and conduct (including ethical conduct) of health care.

Thinking About...

From your own reading, thought and experience, consider what changes there might have been through history in terms of:

- How health has been understood;
- How health has been valued;
- How the ethical purpose and conduct of health care has been understood and evaluated.

The history of trying to understand what health actually *is*

Philosophy (literally, 'love of knowledge') and philosophical questions can be thought of as emerging from the human situation (Warburton, 1999). The 'big' philosophical questions (What is it to be human? How should I live my life?) constitute the traditional territory of the discipline. From the time of the Ancient Greeks, philosophy was the method of rational enquiry into all aspects of human being and existence. Those we would think of today as philosophers (for example, Plato and Aristotle) were in part preoccupied with questions related to the nature of the human body, its function and structure (Turner, 2003: 10). These are the kinds of questions that we would now think of as the prerogative of medicine itself.

Very often (although not always) overshadowing thought about these questions of functioning and so on were religious perspectives. The purpose in asking them was, for many of the ancients, to better understand the laws of God – so-called Natural Philosophy. As human understanding has evolved and progressed over the centuries, rational enquiry has formed and developed through many separate, specific fields and disciplines. One product of the deepening of our knowledge and understanding in this way has been a loosening of the ties between religion and the sciences, and abandoning of the idea of Natural Philosophy. As we have learnt more about our natural world, God has been pushed to the margins of enquiry (and perhaps for many people He is not even there). In this way, investigation related to bodily structure and function, the nature of disease (and in part of 'health', I would argue) has passed from philosophy, frequently overshadowed by theology, to secular medicine with its particular presumptions, values and methods of enquiry. One way of viewing the history of attempts to try to understand what health actually is, then, might be to see it in the context of disciplinary development and movement, with power and control transferring (admittedly over a long period of time) from philosophers and theologians to medics. For the latter, God might not matter very much, if at all.

Thinking About...

If power over the debate about the nature of 'health' itself has shifted from philosophy and religion to secular medicine, consider how might this have changed the way we think about the concept.

The history of health as a *value*

One fairly clear way in which this transfer of power over the health-related debate from the religious to the secular might have had an effect is on how we think about 'health' as a value. In the England of the Middle Ages, Christianity, with its roots in the biblical Old Testament, saw disease as the worldly manifestation of sin. Ill-health represented 'badness' and at least part of the explanation for the bubonic plague that visited England in the sixteenth and seventeenth centuries was provided by a belief that God was punishing sin (a contrary explanation emerging from the more rational traditions of Ancient Greece saw the plague as being caused by corruption of the air and bodily humours) (Thomas, 1997).

If illness and disease were sin, then 'health' was good and consequently an essential moral value. In Protestantism, especially, an important doctrine was that the human body was God-given and therefore we had a fundamental duty to preserve it (Thomas, 1997). Phrases commonly used even now, such as 'Cleanliness is next to Godliness', are among the survivors of a deep and long-lasting belief that the health and hygiene of the body was the external and visible manifestation of the health of the soul.

I have already mentioned Armstrong's analysis of the change in medical beliefs that took place in the late eighteenth century; the move from the belief that disease was caused by 'bad humours' to the idea that specific pathogens were the causative agents of illness. The rapid development in the nineteenth century of the germ theory of disease gave medicine much power, as medical men seemed to demonstrate that they had complete understanding of both how we got sick and what we needed to do to restore ourselves to health. During this period, the nature and value of 'health' became even more synonymous with the 'absence of disease' (Armstrong, 2003). Importantly, in this discussion about the transfer of power from religion to secular medicine, and how it shaped understanding of the value of 'health', the value became free of spiritual (religious) meaning. Indeed, some commentators have suggested that medicine itself has assumed the role of religion in our understanding of the value, and in our trying to acquire more of it. If a historical perspective connects 'disease' with sin and sees 'health' as a moral value that we have a religious duty to pursue, then in our modern, secular age the duty to accept the value in this way and to strive towards it is owed to medicine. In this way, we allow medics all kinds of licence to control and survey us so that we achieve and maintain 'health' (as it is prescribed by medicine) (Armstrong, 1993; Skrabanek and McCormick, 1989).

The history of ethics in *health care*

I suggested before that the Ancient Greeks were founders of the belief that health care (by which we should understand medical practice) was a moral activity. People believed this because health itself was regarded as a moral value. Disease and illness, one way or another, were infractions of the social and moral order. Given this, practical action aiming to tackle these disorders was in general terms morally worthwhile.

This did not mean, of course, that anything medical practitioners did was believed to be acceptable or that practice was always blameless and of value in every case. In particular, physicians (and other health care practitioners) have always had to face questions about the relationship between the practitioner's role as healer, on the one hand, and the rather different one on the other of helping people (when attempts to heal failed) move towards reconciliation with themselves and the idea of their death. (Of course this is also healing, although of another kind.) For the Ancient Greeks, these different roles were both accepted and seen as complementary to each other. The patient sought specific treatment through 'rational' medicine according to the Hippocratic tradition. If this failed, he turned to the holistic model of reconciliation and acceptance, the so-called Asklepian tradition (Randall and Downie, 2006).

Physicians practising in either of these traditions respected the other. The ethical question preoccupying Greek thinkers was primarily that of the nature of 'the good physician'. Who and what was this person like? In the context of this sympathy between the Hippocratic and the Asklepian traditions in the time of the Ancients, answers to this began by trying to understand what it was to be a whole person, with body, soul and mind. The 'good physician' was the one who was able to understand, and respond to, such a person. The route to such understanding was through recognising and trying to develop conceptions of both others and oneself as this kind of person (Haldane, 1986).

> **Q:** The 'good physician' (and by extension, the 'good health care practitioner') is the one who understands the whole person. What problems might there be with this idea of the 'good practitioner'?

One answer to this question lies in the discussions we have already had about historical shifts in the understanding of what health actually is and what kind of value it holds. I have argued that it is possible to show the increasing power, and eventually the overwhelming dominance, of medicine as having the effect of reducing our understanding of 'health' to it being no more than 'the absence of disease'. When the value of health is understood as 'disease absence', the health care work that we most value is the rational, technical, reductionist work in the Hippocratic tradition – that which deals with specific illness and disease. As Randall and Downie (2006) note, the Asklepian tradition has more often than not been left by the wayside in modern medical and health care practice. Given all of this, trying to argue that the 'good practitioner' is the one who attempts to understand and support the development of the 'whole person' (as well as becoming one herself) seems to be going against the grain. In modern times, it could be argued that we value technical competence and technological expertise in health care above everything else.

A Shorter View from History: The Birth of Bioethics

But is this in fact the case? By the mid-twentieth century, the dominance of medicine was at its height, 'health' seemed to be firmly fixed as disease absence, the task of health care was to fix broken bits of bodies and medicine appeared to have assumed the status of a religion. However, at this high tide in medical fortune, it began to be subject to ethical questioning of a kind that had been absent for a long time. As AC Grayling notes: 'Some writers on medical ethics observe that until quite recently the two ethical injunctions by which medical practitioners lived were: do not advertise, and do not have sexual relations with your patients' (Grayling, 2003: 170).

What some have called 'the birth of bioethics' (Jonsen, 1998) changed all that. Within a generation, doctors (and other health care professionals) were being obliged to consider questions of ethics in their basic training and education, as well as at the level of continuing professional development (CPD). Universities were offering a raft of courses to do with medical and health care ethics. Noted medical ethicists were regularly appearing on television and radio (even to the extent of becoming minor 'media stars') to pontificate on questions not so different from those preoccupying the Ancients. Why had all of this happened at a time when medicine's power was apparently at its peak?

Jonsen (1998) offers a useful perspective on reasons for the rise of what he calls 'bioethics', borrowing the definition of the term that is given in the *Encyclopaedia of Bioethics*:

> The systematic study of the moral dimensions – including moral vision, decisions, conduct and policies – of the life sciences and health care, employing a variety of ethical methodologies in an interdisciplinary setting. (Reich, 1995: xix)

While Jonsen is writing mainly about reasons for the rise of the field in the United States, much of what he says is applicable to the rest of the developed world. In the first place, he points to the fact that the decades after the Second World War were ones in which medical science made major advances, still greater than the ones that had preceded this period. Indeed, it's possible to argue that the war itself was the key stimulus to advance, with military-related technology being turned to peaceful use post-1945. In the space of a very few years, medicine assumed a huge capacity to control our lives at their beginnings and endings, as well as at crucial points in between. As technology developed in this exponential way, Jonsen argues that medicine 'left the bedside'. The doctor (the focus was very often on medicine, but it's possible to see medical practice as a kind of emblem for many other branches of health care) turned from a 'folk hero', labouring to bring relief from human suffering, to someone who was rightly subject to doubt and mistrust. He or she had become a 'stranger at the bedside': 'Technology placed the doctor's hands more often on dials than on patients' (Rothman, cited in Cooter, 2000: 257).

From this heightened public mistrust of doctors and other health care workers, now seen as shadowy but highly powerful figures hiding behind mysterious machines that only they could control, there emerged another figure. This was the bioethicist, supposedly appearing to question and submit to examination the practices of health care. However, while it might seem so through a superficial reading of history, this new figure didn't appear by magic. The previous backgrounds of the 'new' bioethicists are also important in understanding why the post-war concern with ethics in health care emerged when it did. The bioethicist came largely from two already-existing disciplines – theology and philosophy.

By the mid-twentieth century, both of these disciplines were under threat. For theology, the expansion of the human mind and possibilities through technology and other means had made us much less likely to believe in God. Yet, paradoxically, as medicine (so it appeared to some) tampered liberally with life and death, we seemed to require explanations for what it meant to be human and lead human lives more than ever before. This was, after all, the period when a disturbed world was trying to come to terms with the horrors of the Holocaust and the first war in history in which civilian (and not only military) casualties had been inflicted on a massive scale. If theologians (academics as well as practical people like priests) couldn't take up the challenge posed by this brave new world, what exactly was their point?

Philosophy, too, faced important questions about its usefulness. I have already talked about the development through history of supposedly rational and objective disciplines and fields of enquiry that had gradually replaced the territory of what was known as Natural Philosophy. Equally, by the middle of the twentieth century, ethics as a branch of philosophy was seen by many to be a discipline that could make little practical difference to peoples' lives. At least in the English-speaking world, the idea of ethics giving any worthwhile guidance on what was right or wrong, or on how we should lead our lives (what is sometimes referred to as normative or 'first order' ethics) had frequently been abandoned. So philosophers also needed a new occupation and direction, and a renewed belief that they could in fact make useful contributions to the practical world. The emerging public mistrust of medicine and health care provided both philosophy and theology, two areas with an almost desperate need for work that was useful and could stand up to scrutiny, with a crucial new direction. It's not too much of an exaggeration to say that doctors and other health care workers, as well as policy makers, came knocking on the doors of theologians and philosophers. And philosophers and theologians, for their own separate reasons, were waiting for the call.

Health Care Professionals and Public Trust

It is possible to argue that bioethics, in drawing together philosophical and theological methodologies, and in its concern to gather interdisciplinary perspectives (from the definition provided by Reich, above) has at least the appearance of a 'novel' field. As I will discuss in the next chapter, this might in fact be a case of the old being dressed up to look like new, of traditional philosophical ethical systems of thinking and methodologies being given a new gloss to make them appear good for disturbing modern times. But whether bioethics is a new invention or simply a re-invention, debates about ethical purpose and practice in health care have of course continued in the half-century or so since what Jonsen describes as its 'birth'.

There are two stimuli to this continued and urgent questioning of the values and ethics of health care and health care professionals, and each is connected to the other. The first is the building in recent years of a coherent theoretical and empirical argument against medicine and health care, at least as they have traditionally been conceived and practised. The second is the actual occurrence of breaches of public trust by health care workers – 'scandals' of one sort or another.

Q.: I am arguing that there are two kinds of stimuli to continuing and often turbulent debate about health care values and ethics:

- The theoretical and empirical argument against 'traditional' medicine and health care;
- The occurrence of medical and health care 'scandals'.

What arguments can you think of against 'traditional' medicine and health care, who developed them and what form do they take? What medical and health care 'scandals' are you aware of that have emerged in recent years? Who was involved, what were their natures and outcomes? What impact have they had on you as a health care worker (or worker-in-training)?

Arguments against 'traditional' medicine and health care

There are two broad kinds of arguments against medicine and health care as traditionally conceived. Some arguments pitch themselves ideologically against (especially) medical practice and try to claim that by virtue of the values and nature of medicine itself, this practice is something that we should be suspicious of or even position ourselves against. There are also other arguments that, through close and extensive empirical work, make the claim that medicine's benefit to the health of the people has been much over-valued. (Thus we should take more seriously the interventions that have been overshadowed by medical practice and yet have *actually* achieved the undoubted improvements in health seen over the last 100 years or so.)

Among the arguments challenging the actual ideology and values of medicine is that of Ivan Illich (1977). Illich argued that far from curing people of disease and restoring them to health, medicine has had the opposite effect; it actually makes people ill, or renders us unable to deal with the disease we already have. It does this, Illich argues, because in the power and control it exerts over individuals and society, it vanquishes our own sense of control and renders us vulnerable to the capricious and harmful treatments of doctors. Illich's theory of **iatrogenesis** (the harmful effects of medicine on society) identifies three particular types of iatrogenic effect. These are: **clinical iatrogenesis** (the harm done through medical treatment); **social iatrogenesis** (the harm done through our individual dependence on medicine as health care 'consumers'); and **structural iatrogenesis** (society's dependence on medicine and the so-called medical model) (Earle, 2007).

Illich's generalised critique has inspired much sociological attention towards the practices of medicine. In particular, attention has been turned to the ways that it has 'medicalised' what are in fact normal, healthy events, such as pregnancy and childbirth. Medicine has also (wrongly) attempted to 'treat' things that should be seen simply as part of the human condition. For example, it has turned sadness, something that we will all feel at some points in our lives, into the clinical and supposedly treatable condition of 'depression' (Earle, 2007).

Other ideological critiques include that of the lawyer and philosopher Ian Kennedy. In a series of BBC Reith lectures in 1981, which eventually became his book, *The Unmasking of Medicine* (Kennedy, 1981), he argued broadly that medicine focuses on the disease process to the exclusion of the actual patient herself.

The second kind of argument against the traditions and practice of health care, as I have said, is supposedly founded on empirical evidence that in fact medicine has had little to do with health improvement in Western societies. An important example of this kind of argument is that developed by Thomas McKeown, who was a professor of social medicine at Birmingham University and published his book, *The Role of Medicine* in 1976 (McKeown, 1976). Using especially the example of tuberculosis (TB) decline in England and Wales, he argued that the falling death rate in these countries since 1870 was largely the result of improvements in nutrition and sanitation, which had the effect of making people more resistant to disease. As a consequence, death rates decreased although he argued that this had *relatively* little to do with medicine.

Since its publication, McKeown's argument has been heavily criticised, not least because of its strong reliance on statistics and his comparative neglect of the 'rich historical context' of the period during which death rates fell (Hardy, 2001: 10). However, the very fact and time of its publication gave it significance. As I have already described, this was the same time that Illich (and later Kennedy) were publishing their own ideological critiques of 'traditional' medicine and health care. The fact that McKeown joined the chorus gave still more weight to the general social doubt emerging in the mid-1970s about the position of medicine, especially as he was actually a medic himself. Indeed, it is possible to directly link these separate but nevertheless connected challenges to medical authority to movements that can be seen as offering an alternative to the narrow 'medical model', for example, the so-called New Public Health (Duncan, 2004).

Medical and health care 'scandals'

These theoretical and empirical attacks against medicine and health care, at least as they have been traditionally conceived, have also been strengthened by the seemingly endless succession of health care 'scandals' that have been uncovered in relatively recent times. Of course we have to doubt and mistrust doctors and other health care workers, some people would say, just look at what they are actually *doing*! During recent years, we have only to think of, for example, the mass-murdering GP Harold Shipman or the paediatric nurse and child-murderer Beverley Allitt. Then there are the Bristol Heart Babies' surgeons, the gynaecologist Rodney Ledward, who mis-operated on many women, and the case of illicit organ retention at Alder Hey Children's Hospital. This is not to mention the many other less well-known and less reported cases where professionals have breached the trust of their patients or clients (Revill, 2006a).

Q: What exactly do you know about any or all of the 'scandals' I have just mentioned? How did you gather your knowledge? How did you react when you first heard about events? Write down your memory of thoughts and reactions at the time.

The purpose of these particular questions is to try to draw out the importance of these 'scandals' in contributing to the current build up of alarm about health care professionals in our society. Each of the 'scandals' that I have mentioned has culminated in an inquiry into what went wrong and why (see, for example, Kennedy (2001) and Smith (2002, 2003)). Such inquiries very often form a focus for renewed media attention on the case concerned (some months or even more after the events themselves) and thus provide us with an extended opportunity to form or review our thoughts and beliefs about what happened and why. (The opportunity is extended because coverage of inquiries very often lasts for weeks and perhaps months.) As Stanley and Manthorpe (2004) argue, inquiries provoke huge interest. They become narratives filled with human drama and action. Indeed, their published versions sometimes have titles that are more reminiscent of detective novels or thrillers than sober public investigations. For example, part of the title of Dame Janet Smith's first report into the Shipman case was 'Death Disguised'. They gather much of their dramatic tension from the fact that we know already what has happened, since the events they are trying to piece together and understand would have happened months or possibly years before. So we are able not only to see the story unfolding, but also to make continuous and then final ethical judgements about the actors in the narrative. Inquiries into health care 'scandals' therefore have the capacity to promote not only moral judgement, but also moral 'panic' (Stanley and Manthorpe, 2004: 2–3). Their impact on our conscious and subconscious assessment of the 'trustworthiness' of health care professionals is substantial.

Of course I am not trying to suggest that we shouldn't thoroughly investigate when things go wrong in medical and health care; nor that the matters examined by inquiries are somehow trivial. They are certainly not. They have had dramatic effects and repercussions on the lives of many people, most often when those people were in highly vulnerable circumstances. This is a hugely important part of the reason why we need to investigate what went wrong and why. But by virtue of the terrible human tragedies from which inquiries into medical and health care 'scandals' emerge, and by virtue of the nature and form of the inquiries themselves, we are left with events and stories of events that provide vivid reminders of why we should doubt health care professionals.

Conclusion: Bioethics, Health Care Professionals and the 'Gap in Trust'

This chapter has offered some historical perspectives on the place of talk about values and ethics in health care. I have argued that questions of ethics and values applied to the fields of health and health care have long been asked, and attempts to answer them have much deeper roots than the contemporary phenomenon of 'bioethics'. However, there are tangible reasons why bioethics (health care ethics) has in recent times taken such an important place in health care practice and teaching. It is possible to point especially to the rise of technology applied to medicine and health care and the blurring of the traditional boundaries of life, death and what it means to be human itself in explaining its importance. Technological advance has seemingly converted doctors and health care workers generally from people of compassion and sympathy into shadowy figures hiding behind machines. Given this, our moral concern is entirely understandable.

While this has been happening (and as one consequence of it), opponents of medicine and health care have been developing powerful critiques of practice in the fields. Belief in the once all-powerful 'medical model' has diminished. At the same time, we have been more willing to question practices and, when things go wrong, to probe more thoroughly into why this has happened. The results of this probing are often uncomfortable. While Dr Shipman and Beverley Allitt, say, murdered by themselves, and certainly in Allitt's case there was identifiable mental illness (Hart, 2004), this fails to explain *why* they were able to kill in the first place. And in the case of the Bristol Heart Babies (along with many others), the very systems that were supposed to protect the vulnerable failed to work (Kennedy, 2001).

All this has led to the point where society is experiencing a 'gap in trust' between the people who seek the services of professionals to keep them healthy or restore them to health and the professionals who 'profess' (Koehn, 1994) to be able to offer such help. If our current concern with health care ethics has emerged at least partly because of the recent historical and contemporary context that I have described, then it seems reasonable to ask whether and how it can meet the challenge posed by this 'gap in trust'. The challenge applies not just in the 'big cases' of Shipman, Bristol, Alder Hey, and so on. It is equally important (I would argue more so) to try to meet the challenge in relation to the everyday encounters of *all* health care professionals, whether they are involved in caring for or treating people who are sick, or are concerned with helping individuals or communities to seek and maintain health. How this might be done and what resources ethics can provide to help with the task forms the content for much of the rest of this book.

Chapter Summary

In this chapter, I have:

- Argued that philosophical and ethical thinking related to health care is a complex interplay between philosophers and the society of which they are part;
- Outlined the long history of the philosophical and ethical interest in health care;
- Argued that, one way or another, through all of this long history, 'health' has always been seen as a moral value, and health care as a moral activity;
- Argued that scientific and social advances from the mid-twentieth century onwards were largely responsible for the emergence of the field of 'bioethics';
- Explained that the current 'gap in trust' between health care professionals and patients or clients requires the attention of bioethics because this is what gave 'birth' to the field in the first place.

Further Reading

Porter, R (1999). *The Greatest Benefit to Mankind*. London: HarperCollins. This is a brilliant account of the historical development of medicine, against which it is possible to plot changing attitudes and values among those affected by or practising it.

Jonsen, AR (1998). *The Birth of Bioethics*. Oxford: Oxford University Press. Jonsen writes a history of how bioethics developed. It is made all the more useful by the fact that he himself was one of its pioneers.

4

ETHICAL THINKING: OBLIGATIONS AND CONSEQUENCES

Learning Outcomes

By the end of this chapter, you should be able to:

○ Describe and discuss a theory of ethics based on a consideration of *obligation* or *duty*;
○ Describe and discuss a theory of ethics based on a consideration of the *consequences* of action;
○ Identify, describe and discuss both problems and possibilities attached to each of these kinds of theory in the practical health care context;
○ Offer a reasoned view on the worth of these theories to those working in health care.

Introduction

I argued in Chapter 2 that it is reasonable to see ethics as concerning how we ought to act in general, and as trying to determine what is of value to us and why. This led in turn to the idea of potentially contrasting approaches in ethical thinking. On the one hand, we might be interested in trying to work out what we should always generally try to do, regardless of the consequences of our actions. We might reasonably talk of ethics in this sense as being about attempts to frame generalised **obligations** or **duties** for action (as well as proposing justifications for these obligations). On the other hand, if we are interested in the nature of **values** and what we should be promoting as valuable, we might frame our ethical thinking around the **consequences** of action instead of around fixed obligations. After all, if we are concerned to produce more of something that we consider to be valuable, our main focus will be on what we need to do and how we should act in order to ensure the best chance that more of this value will be produced.

There is not necessarily always a conflict between these two different ways of seeing ethics. It is possible to take the view that one of our most important general obligations is to try to act so that what we do is most likely to produce more of what we believe to be valuable. In this way, obligations and values are reconciled. But such a view hides a tension that is very often present in our thoughts about what we should do. There will often be times when what we feel we should do (our sense of obligation or duty) is unlikely to lead to the best outcome (the production of most value).

> Q: Can you think of a situation (ideally from your own practice or potential practice in health care) in which there has been, or is likely to be, a conflict between what you think you ought to do and what is likely to produce 'the best result'? Make a note of your example.

One of my main claims in this chapter is that while there is not necessarily always conflict between obligations and consequences, in practice there often is. If we are to understand the nature of this conflict, and how it might impact on our own health care practice, then we need to ask three questions:

- What kinds of arguments have philosophers developed for the importance of obligations, on the one hand, and consequences, on the other, as being at the ethical root of our action?
- Why have these arguments been developed?
- How do they affect our own thinking and practice?

These questions draw us into two important traditions of ethical thinking: **deontology** (what we might call the ethics of obligation or duty) and **consequentialism** (the ethics of consequences). My plan in this chapter is to describe and discuss these two different traditions. Building on the arguments of the last chapter, though, I also want to connect these traditions to the times in which they were developed. If, as I have argued, philosophy and philosophers are products of their social times, then reasons for particular philosophical concerns become more understandable. This in turn makes the whole philosophical project itself more understandable and meaningful. My claim now is that deontological and consequentialist traditions can at least in part be better understood by considering the times in which their key protagonists developed them.

How Should We Act? What is Valuable?

These questions lie at the heart of projects of ethics. They are of key relevance to both the ethicist advocating deontology and the ethicist who proposes consequentialism. This is perhaps how each of them would respond to the questions:

- The deontologist would say that we should always act according to the moral obligations or duties that we believe ourselves to have. Value lies in our always acting in this way. For example, I should always tell the truth, and value most properly lies in my absolute commitment to truth-telling (or whatever other obligations I believe myself to have).
- The consequentialist would argue that we should always act in such a way that the action concerned is likely to produce the best possible consequences. Our motivation in acting should always be to produce more of what we believe to be valuable. Probably, the most well-known consequentialist theory is **utilitarianism**, which proposes we should always act so that we produce the greatest possible happiness for the greatest number of people (Mill, 1962). For the utilitarian, then, the valuable is happiness and its maximisation.

I've already suggested that there might well be some occasions where the concerns of the deontologist, on the one hand, and the consequentialist, on the other, may meet quite happily. For example, I may commit myself to action (feel myself to have a moral obligation to act) only when acting will produce worthwhile consequences. But this attempt to draw obligations and consequences together presents some difficulties.

Q. What difficulties might there be in attempting to draw thoughts about obligations and thoughts about consequences together in this kind of way? You might be helped in answering this question by returning to the example you generated just before of the difficult situation in which there seemed to be a conflict between what you felt you ought to do and what action was likely to have the best consequences.

A major difficulty in drawing together obligations and consequences in this way might be that it provides us with no firm and practical basis for action. If I am constantly thinking about what I should be doing next in order to produce the best consequences, then my moral compass will always be changing. In this situation, it would be a good idea for me to tell the truth; in that one, it would probably be better for me to lie. I might start to feel a bit chameleon-like. An obligation 'to produce the best possible consequences' seems just too vague; surely I should simply do my best to tell the truth as often as I possibly can? Equally though, it doesn't seem possible to avoid thought about the consequences of our actions altogether. Blindly telling the truth without any care for what will happen is likely to lead to at least some difficult consequences on some occasions. So the drawing together of deontology (obligation ethics) and consequentialism (ethics based on thought of consequences) seems problematic. At the very least, on the basic assessment made so far, it seems to have the potential to lead us, possibly quite often, towards moral ambiguity and doubt.

A Context, Situation and Example for Debates about Obligations and Consequences

Whenever we think about obligations (duties) and consequences, we are almost always thinking of these things in relation to a particular context or situation and probably a specific example. It would be very hard for me to say, 'I have an obligation to tell the truth' without ever thinking of contexts and circumstances in which truth-telling would be a good thing to do (or alternatively, where it might result in potential problems). Equally, it would be difficult to imagine an interest in consequences that wasn't ever related to thought about the consequences of a *particular* situation or a *specific* example (and the value or otherwise of those consequences occurring). This is not to assert that we can't think generally about the kinds of obligations we might have, or about the broad sorts of consequences we might want to see resulting from what we do; nor that we can't want everybody to hold those values or obligations. Indeed, there is an argument in philosophy that unless we can wish for general application of an obligation or a value, then that obligation or value is not a moral one. This is sometimes referred to as the requirement for moral obligations or values to be **generalisable**. That is to say, if I hold truth-telling (for example) to be a moral obligation, then everybody else should do so too (Lacey, 1976).

However, the key point is that unless I can think of a situation or context in which a particular obligation or value has relevance, and more often than not a specific example, then we need to question the point of thinking about that obligation or value in the first place. In other words, we develop and practise our ethical thinking in 'real world' contexts and situations, and by reference to examples we have experienced or can imagine. This means that in order properly to understand the worth of (and the problems with) particular theories of ethics, we have to see how they might apply in the world.

The context for us, of course, is contemporary health care. The particular situation and example that I want to use to tease out some of the problems and possibilities with deontological and consequentialist theories relate to a subject I discussed in Chapter 1. This is the issue of childhood obesity.

Example

In Chapter 1, I used the case of bariatric surgery in later childhood to begin unpacking some of the problems connected to the issue of obesity in children. The issue has major political significance, with it sometimes seeming that hardly a day goes by without media coverage of what appears increasingly to be portrayed as an 'epidemic', a 'ticking time bomb', containing disastrous future levels of morbidity and mortality. The bariatric surgery case raised lots of questions

(Continued)

(Continued)

to do with resource allocation, rights and responsibilities. Should we be siphoning off scarce NHS money to pay for surgery for teenagers who have eaten themselves into the ground? But then surely we should do what we can to prevent the miserable lives that obesity leads to? Whose responsibility is it that children have become fat in the first place? Is it their own, or their parents, or broader society? Is it right to advocate 'thinness' almost as a moral state, at the same time presenting obesity as a fall from grace and obese people as very nearly social outcasts?

It is against this broad context and situation that the following specific example emerges. Julie Seale is a practice nurse working in a medium-sized general practice in an outer suburb of London. The area that the practice serves is generally quite affluent, but it also contains two council estates with relatively high levels of deprivation. The practice is quite proactive on health promotion and public health issues, and at the moment is particularly concerned about obesity. One of the partners, Dr Williams, is also a governor at a local primary school where she has been discussing with the head teacher the idea of a joint approach on the part of the practice and the school with regard to childhood obesity. The plan is that the school will run a number of sessions for the children on 'healthy eating', which will involve some of the practice staff, including Julie. A letter to be sent to each child's home before the sessions begin will inform parents or carers about what is happening. A follow-up letter after the sessions will invite the carers or parents to contact the practice for further information and advice about family eating patterns, diet, and so on.

Julie will be responsible for managing any follow-up on behalf of the practice. As she is also currently taking a short course on health care ethics at the local university, she is interested in thinking about the moral implications of the intervention. Can it be justified through consideration of *obligations* that she (or others in the practice) might have, or through thought about its *consequences* (or through both)?

Almost at the very beginning of this book, I used the dramatic case of Dr Irwin and Mrs Murphy to provide one of the illustrations for my claim that consideration of values and ethics is fundamental to those involved in health care. But I have tried to stress since then that values and ethics do not permeate only this sort of highly charged example. They also run through apparently much less dramatic examples, including this one, which is very likely to feature in the practice of many involved in health care (Leith, 2007). My purpose in choosing the example of Julie Seale is in part to further underline the ethical problematic of 'ordinary' health care. As I will argue now, we can relate this health promotion example as easily to the major Western ethical traditions that I have begun to identify as we can the problems that emerge in acute health care. These traditions can offer as much (or possibly as little) help to Julie as they can to those thinking about Dr Irwin and Mrs Murphy.

It's All about What *I Must* Do: Deontological Ethics

Let's begin by thinking in some more detail about deontology – the ethics of obligation, or duty. One of the central (and highly difficult) tasks for the deontologist – the philosopher attempting to establish duty as the moral ground of our action – is to argue for *why* this should be the case, as well as *exactly what sort of* duties we should hold.

> Q: •Why do you think duty should form the ethical basis for our action, and •what sorts of duties ought we to hold? Note down your response.

One of the reasons that you might have come up with for the importance of duty in deciding how to act is that certain kinds of relationships (for example, parents and children, or professionals and clients) actually *entail* duties. Parents have a duty to look after their offspring. We could also argue that when a certain point is reached in life, this duty is reversed. Professionals (say, social workers or nurses) have a duty to care for their clients or patients. We could argue that these separate examples are rather different from each other. Professional obligations emerge at least in part from things like written contracts of employment, whereas this is unlikely to be so in the case of parents and children. (Although there are such things as 'Parenting Agreements', which are sometimes applied in cases of dispute about care of children affected by separation and divorce.) In general, though, it would be hard to dispute that many people are bound to others through duties and obligations, whether written or unwritten. However, there are problems with this response to the question that I've posed:

- It only covers *certain kinds of relationships*, whereas the question asked for reasons why duty should form the basis for all our action;
- Even within these kinds of relationships, where we believe that we have certain sorts of duty, the nature of the duty is likely to be both prescribed and circumscribed. Would we be happy, say, that a nurse who 'did his duty' by following his contract of employment to the letter (always starting and finishing exactly on time, and so on) was acting *ethically*? This conception of 'duty' seems narrow against the more expansive ideas that we tend to have about what constitutes genuinely moral action.

Given these doubts, we might want to argue the following. For an ethics of duty to be acceptable as a basis for all action, it has to be both generally applicable (and not just within some kinds of relationships). It should also not be (or at least not unduly) limited and circumscribed. As I will discuss shortly, meeting both of these criteria might be very difficult.

The father of duty-based theories of ethics is almost universally agreed to be the Prussian philosopher Immanuel Kant (1724–1804). Kant is also often regarded as the greatest of modern philosophers (Russell, 1979). His life was an academic and unremarkable one; it is said that people used to set their watches according to when they saw him pass by their houses on his daily constitutional! (Russell, 1979: 678.) But Kant was working at the time of the Enlightenment, the period that began in the eighteenth century and was characterised by the rich and powerful burgeoning of knowledge and understanding – especially of scientific knowledge. This rapid expansion of the territory of scientific explanation led to the belief that the use of reason alone could help us explain and deal with all aspects of the world. Advances in medicine and in the physical and biological sciences at this time took on the character of revolutions. It must have appeared as if a veil was being drawn back after a long period of darkness to expose the light of discovery and progress. Against all this, Kant's project was to apply reason to solve the great problems of philosophy, including problems of ethics.

The focus on **reason** in Kant's arguments has led philosophers to characterise them as *a priori*. An argument is *a priori* if it is constructed independently of experience, through the use of processes of reason and deduction. Such arguments contrast with those that depend on experience (**empirical** arguments) for their formation and strength (Duncan, 2007). Kant's general view is that *a priori* knowledge and reason form the strongest (in fact the only possible) basis for our ethical decision-making.

Thinking About...

The distinction between *a priori* and non-*a priori* argument is important in philosophy. It is a difficult distinction, however, and worth spending some time thinking about, especially as it seems to be the case that most of the arguments we use in everyday life employ calls to experience in some way to support them. For example, suppose my family asks me to give them an argument as to why we should all go on holiday by train next year. Quite possibly, my argument will be based at least in part on direct experience; the year before last we went on holiday by train and it was an enjoyable and comfortable experience, much more so than last year's holiday-by-car disaster. But imagine that our family had never been on holiday by train before. If this were the case, I would have to develop an argument for why we should do this, without reference to any prior experience *of our family having travelled on holiday together by train*. Of course, in developing that argument I might be relying on other kinds of experiences (for example, journeys that I have taken by myself by train and where I have experienced the comfort of train travel). Essentially, however, my argument will be *a priori* because it does not depend on or make reference to an exactly analogous experience – our family simply doesn't have one.

My example of the family holiday by train exposes a central difficulty in *a priori* argument. It was necessary for me to quite finely distinguish that it was such because we had never had that *particular* experience before. However, imagination, *vicarious example* and *broadly similar* situations would probably have played a part as I developed my case. The task that Kant sets himself in his argument for duty as the basis of action is to try to move from the *a priori*-experience mix of many of our arguments to one that works through reason alone.

Duty as the moral basis for action

So what is the nature of this argument through reason alone? Kant sets it out in a work rather dauntingly entitled *Groundwork of the Metaphysic of Morals* (Paton, 1948). The argument begins with the claim that there is only one thing that is good in itself, and that is a **good will**. There are many other things that are good in some circumstances, but only a good will is good under all circumstances. A good will is not demonstrated by acting out of inclination, or worse still out of self-interest. These motivations for action are likely to lead at least sometimes (possibly often) to ethical difficulties. The proper motivation for our action is **duty**, and acting for the sake of duty is the proper expression of good will.

Moreover, acting for duty's sake is an expression of reason. If we act through self-interest or inclination (without proper consideration of duty), then we are likely to be faced with harmful or chaotic results. Only acting out of duty will yield reasonable outcomes. For example, imagine that I only told the truth when it suited me to do so. This would quickly result in people not knowing whether to trust me in a given situation. On the other hand, if I held truth-telling as a duty, then others' trust in me would be consistent and constant. The first ground for my actions – self-interest – cannot possibly be based on reason because if everybody acted in this way, the world would soon grind to a halt, with nobody trusting anybody else. The second ground – duty – is obviously based on rationality and reason because we know that holding truth-telling as constant is likely to serve humanity much better. We owe it to each other to express good will through acting for the sake of duty precisely because we are all rational beings most properly guided by reason rather than impulse or instinct. This in turn leads to Kant's formulation of what is called the 'categorical imperative': 'Act only on that maxim through which you can at the same time will that it should become a universal law' (Paton, 1948: 29). I cannot wish for anything to be a principle for action unless it applies to everybody. Continuing with the lying example, it couldn't possibly be the case that I would want lying to assume the status of a universal law because the results of this would be completely adverse, not simply to me but to all my fellows.

Kant's argument for duty as the ethical basis for action is grounded, we can now see, on a number of *a priori* statements or judgements. (That is to say, he is constructing them as truths in themselves, without reference to experience.) The judgements are:

- A good will is the only thing good in itself;
- The proper demonstration of a good will is acting for the sake of duty;
- Acting for duty's sake is an expression of reason;
- We are bound to each other as rational human beings to act for the sake of duty.

Yet we have to live in the real world of senses and experience. The key question for practical people, such as health care workers, is to try to establish what are the effects of this *a priori* argument on their own practical reality. Does it make sense? Does it help? To think about these kinds of questions, we will return to Julie Seale and the issue of childhood obesity.

Duty in the context of the childhood obesity example

Kant's argument does not list or even hint at particular duties that we should hold (Cottingham, 2008). What it does is to provide a **ground** for the essential importance of duty in our ethical thinking. (Duty is the proper expression of reason in action, and we cannot conceive of action as ethical unless we can also will that everybody else should act in the same way.) But bearing in mind the truth-telling and lying example above, it seems, at least initially, that it wouldn't be so difficult to come up with duties or obligations that Julie Seale might feel she has in the context of the example.

Q.•What kinds of duties or obligations do you think Julie might feel she has as
 •she begins work on the 'healthy eating' intervention? List your responses.

The kinds of things that you might have come up with perhaps include the following:

- A duty to respect the beliefs, wishes and situations of the parents and children involved in the intervention;
- A duty to tell the truth about what is happening and what the outcomes are likely to be;
- A duty to apply the resources available for the intervention in a fair and equitable way.

You may of course have used different expressions. For example, you could have referred to a generalised 'duty of care'. However, it's probably the case that my expression of the duties Julie feels she has resonates with yours to at least some degree, even if it doesn't match exactly with what you might have written down. To this extent, we could suggest that a Kantian framework, or ground, for moral action has justifications. I might well be able to will that all these possible duties are universally held, or at least health care workers hold them universally. Certainly, it seems odd to argue that health care workers don't have these kinds of duties or obligations (Gillon, 1990). If I were to claim that health care workers had obligations to be profligate with resources, to go around concealing the truth from patients or clients and to disregard their wishes and interests, I would most likely be thought mad.

What we seem to be saying is that all health care workers should hold the duties listed above (or duties that are very similar). This statement matches with Kant's ground because we can see that we would want to will these duties for those working in health care. There is, I would agree, the question as to whether the duties are **universalisable** to all, whether health care workers or not. It would seem strange to claim that lay people have a duty in relation to the allocation of scarce health care resources. But I think this question can be answered in two ways:

- It may be sufficient to argue for universalisability to health care workers alone. After all, common sense seems to tell us that those working in health care do indeed have particular obligations, such as those relating to resource use. I will explore this idea more fully in later chapters.
- Even if we doubt this and believe that the specificity of the obligations to health care workers goes against Kant's ground of universal willing, we can say that we all (health care workers or not) hold similar sorts of obligations. If I am not working in health care, then obviously I don't have a duty in relation to the *application* of resources, but I do have one with regard to their *receipt*. For example, I shouldn't wantonly go around getting access to services and treatment that I don't really need. So with a bit more care, we could frame a duty for proper application and use of scarce resources that is actually properly universalisable – for both lay people and those working in health care.

All of this might lead us to believe that there are duties that we can will for everyone, and so that correspond to Kant's ground for the morality of action. This is the thread of Julie's thought as she considers the work with the primary school, its pupils, parents and teachers. In fact, she is inclined to think that all health care workers should generally have these kinds of obligations. However, there are two questions that nag at her:

- Should all those working in health care have these obligations *all the time and in every circumstance*?
- Should they all have these obligations *to all patients or clients in equal measure*?

Julie's worries have been prompted by more detailed exploration of the potential implications contained within the list of duties described above. Take the first one:

- A duty to respect the beliefs, wishes and situations of the parents and children involved in the intervention.

Generally speaking, this might be quite a reasonable duty to uphold in this circumstance. But in fact it is quite complex. In the first place, two sets of people are involved – parents and children. Do we owe parents, on the one hand, and children, on the other, the same kind and same amount of respect? Some would argue that children, by virtue of their developing mental awareness and capacity, require guidance and control until they reach a certain age, regarded by the law at least as the age of majority (18 in the UK context). Indeed, many would see this kind of 'shaping' as a key purpose of education (Carr, 2003).

This leads to the idea that there are limits to the degree to which we can allow children to do exactly what they want whenever they want to. Teachers and parents, and others with responsibility for the welfare of children, step in when they see risk or likely adverse results of a child's behaviour. Freedom is limited out of interests for the child's protection. In this case, would Julie be able to sit by as a child continued with grossly unhealthy eating habits? (For that matter, would parents and teachers be able to do so?) By its nature, the intervention aims to promote behaviour change if necessary and this may well result in conflict in some cases. There may then be circumstances in which *some* beliefs and wishes are respected more than are others.

This leads to the second complexity within the duty. It's relatively easy to imagine less respect being paid to a child who wants to eat unhealthy food all the time, and their being subject to degrees of pressure to make the 'right' food choices. (Of course, this wouldn't involve sitting them down and forcing them to eat a plate of greens; it would probably be done in more subtle but certainly still controlling ways, such as having nothing other than healthy 'options' available on the school canteen menu.) But can we pay equal respect to all of the variety of wishes and beliefs that *parents* involved with the intervention might have? What if one of the effects of the intervention is to draw a response from a number of parents who complain that their children are being 'brain-washed with too many ideas' and that the families concerned are quite happy with their current eating behaviour? This is more or less likely to be 'unhealthy' in health care professional terms, but should Julie make this clear to an irate parent turning up at the surgery? Should she try to persuade them to think again? If such an incident happened, and she was to do this, then there's no doubt that limits would have been placed on the degree to which the parent's beliefs and wishes had been respected. We might see this as a (probably very weak) form of what philosophers often call **paternalism** (Gorovitz, 1985). This is an attempt to place limits on the freedom of adults in the way that we feel often justified in doing so with children.

Julie has doubts about the extent of the second duty as well:

- A duty to tell the truth about what is happening and what the outcomes are likely to be.

The problem for her is not truth-telling as a general principle; she has no doubt of her duty to be as honest as possible with patients or clients. The difficulty lies in both how much truth she is *able* to convey and how much it is *best* to do so. In Chapter 1, we identified childhood obesity as a complex problem with many different strands (NHS Centre for Reviews and Dissemination, 2002). In Julie's potential talks with both children and parents, just how much of this complexity should she try to convey? How much is it desirable to do so? Would it be right, for example, if she made it clear that attempts at healthy eating require careful navigation through a society where a greater premium is often placed on things like convenience and profit than it is on health? For some, this level of honesty might be acceptable. For others, it might be less so. At the very least, telling the truth in this way requires careful thought, especially with people who don't necessarily have the skills and resources in place at the moment to cope with the many pressures *against* healthy eating. This is not to say that the complexities shouldn't be explained. However, if we are to avoid alarming such 'vulnerable' people, or promoting feelings of helplessness, this level of truth-telling will have to go hand in hand with efforts to provide them with the necessary resources and to teach them appropriate skills. These may not always be present.

Nor is the third duty that Julie identified unproblematic:

- A duty to apply the resources available for the intervention in a fair and equitable way.

As I have described, the geographical area that Julie works in is generally affluent but there are some pockets of deprivation. There is, as we know, a substantial body of empirical work that clearly sets out the case for social and economic deprivation causing ill-health and making it harder for somebody to maintain their levels of health (see, for example, Townsend et al., 1988; Wilkinson, 2005). Given this knowledge, along with understanding of her own context, Julie is faced with a difficulty. Dr Williams and the school have decided that the intervention should be applied equally to all the children, and families should have equal access to any follow-up that they wish. Practically, this makes a lot of sense; it would be hard to differentiate so that, say, only children and families coming from a particular part of the school catchment area came to the 'healthy eating' sessions, or got access to the follow-up advice. Not only would it be practically hard, it would also be tantamount to pointing a finger at these families and saying, 'You're *different* – you need our help.'

On the other hand, Julie is well aware of the very strong arguments for the existence of inequalities, and also of what is known as 'the inverse care law' (Tudor Hart, 1971). This is the uncomfortable principle for health services that those people who have least need of health care workers' attentions and skills are most likely to get them. From her daily experience, she comes across what she calls 'the middle-class worried well', who generally speaking get what they want from the practice. At the same time, she sees single parents on low incomes struggling to cope with their difficult circumstances and the impact that this has on their own and their families' health. So this duty prompts in Julie's mind a range of questions about whether resources are indeed being applied fairly and equitably here, whether she should challenge their application and what the results of any challenge might be.

Whether or not you generally agree with the problems that I have argued for in relation to these duties, perhaps the nub of the difficulty lies in the fact that it is possible to dispute their nature, and what they suggest or imply. This returns us to the purpose of the deontological project. What Kant (and other deontologists) are trying to do is to develop and defend a ground for our actions. Kant's *a priori* argument initially sounds appealing. Acting for the sake of duty is action based on reason; we should only act when we can properly will that this duty and action is universally applicable. But the argument is *a priori*, independent of experience. The example of Julie and the healthy eating intervention has shown that while we might agree with Kant's ground for action, individual circumstances make it hard to frame particular duties that cannot be contested, or disagreed about. The ground could be generally applicable (and not just within some kinds of relationships), but the nature of particular duties is likely to be subject to contest and dispute according to circumstance. And if this is the case, what is the point of having the kind of ground for ethical action that Kant proposes? It seems that all we might be able to say is something like the following:

- I can act out of duty and will my action for all others *provided that* the circumstances they face make the action in that case an ethical one.

This conclusion seems quite a long way from the universal applicability of duty that the deontologist is arguing for. If we cannot say (at least without argument) what duties count in what circumstances, how can we accept without reservation an ethics based solely on considerations of duty?

It's What Happens that Counts: Consequentialist Ethics

This leads us to thoughts of what other considerations might be relevant to the framing of an action in ethical terms. There is an important philosophical tradition concerned with developing the idea that considering the **consequences** of actions should lie at the heart of our moral thinking. The English philosopher Jeremy Bentham (1748–1832) is often regarded as the first major consequentialist thinker. Probably the best known, however, is John Stuart Mill (1806–73).

Bentham, to an extent, and Mill certainly were working yet again during a period of major historical and social change. The early to mid-nineteenth century saw the development of the Industrial Revolution, first in the United Kingdom and then spreading to many other European countries. Raw materials were used, and goods produced, on scales never seen previously. Mines and factories sprang up. Ports, canals and railways were developed to carry goods from place to place and country to country. There were dramatic patterns of migration from the countryside to towns and cities, which rapidly grew in population, a trend that was to continue throughout the nineteenth century and change Britain from a rural to an essentially urban society (Hardy, 2001).

An important effect of these changes was that the relationship between individuals and the communities and societies in which they lived altered dramatically. Whereas for most, prior to the onset of industrialisation, there had been a dependence on neighbours and others in small communities, now many relied heavily on people they had never seen. Remote employers paid their wages, distant politicians increasingly laid down laws that regulated their lives, organisations that were well removed provided utilities such as water, sewage, gas and, later, electricity. (Or perhaps they failed to do so, with disastrous consequences for large numbers of the population.) The action or inaction of a few, or even just one person, could now affect many. A central question in this new world was: How should one act?

Consideration of consequences as the moral basis for action

Probably the most famous statement of consequentialist thought is contained in JS Mill's *Utilitarianism* (Mill, 1962), originally published in 1861. Contrary to the suggestion of its name, Mill's work does not argue that we should seek only the useful, but rather that we should pursue the good in itself. But what forms the good? The principle at the heart of utilitarianism is this:

> The creed which accepts the foundation of morals, Utility, or the Greatest Happiness Principle, holds that actions are right in proportion as they tend to promote happiness, wrong as they tend to produce the reverse of happiness. By happiness is intended pleasure, and the absence of pain; by unhappiness, pain, and the privation of pleasure. (Mill, 1962: 257)

What should guide my actions, then, is a concern that they produce the best possible consequences in terms of an increase in happiness. Pleasure, the product of happiness, is the only reasonable (ethical) end of action. The sole kind of action we can view as ethical is that which, as a consequence of us performing it, will produce happiness and therefore pleasure. (In fact, utilitarianism, in at least some of its forms, holds that for an action to be regarded as good (ethical) it doesn't necessarily have to be performed with *good intentions*, but only to produce *good effects*.)

Q.•What do you think are the benefits and drawbacks attached to utilitarianism, the ethical theory that places consequences at the heart of action and views acts as ethical to the extent that they produce happiness and pleasure?

Consequentialism and utilitarianism are sometimes referred to as **teleological** theories of ethics. What this means is that we only have obligations or duties in so far as they lead to the production of valuable ends. Teleological theories offer an apparent contrast to deontology. As I have argued, deontological theory asserts that duty exists independently of thought about what value might be produced through acting. One difficulty with promoting this contrast as absolute is that it seems strange, in a practical sense, completely to disengage actions and consequences from one another (Lacey, 1976). Perhaps the most sensible way to see the distinction between a deontological theory of ethics, such as Kant's, on the one hand, and utilitarianism on the other is in terms of the kind of emphasis that each places on the nature of value and how it is produced:

- For the deontologist, the value of an action lies mainly (or even completely) in it being the performance of duty;
- For the consequentialist, the value of an action rests mainly or wholly in the extent to which it produces goods.

The task facing Julie Seale now is to try to work out whether a shift in emphasis from duty to consequences helps her ethical assessment of the healthy eating intervention.

Thinking about the consequences in the context of the childhood obesity example

At least to begin with, putting consequences closer to the heart of ethical consideration provides Julie with some relief! She was rather daunted by the difficulties facing her as she tried to frame her ethical assessment solely in terms of obligation or duty. Thinking about the value of an action in terms of what is likely to be produced by undertaking it seems quite reasonable and in line with everyday thinking. Not only that, the maximisation of happiness, according to the utilitarian rubric, also seems a reasonable objective for her and, she thinks, for many others involved in health care. It would be quite odd to approach health care work as indifferent to the levels of happiness you might be helping to produce, or to work with a dominant alternative rubric – for example, the production of more economic efficiency (although of course this might form *part of* an approach). If Julie, along with the other practice staff and those working at the school, engages in the intervention carefully and conscientiously, she thinks it is highly likely that value will be produced. Children and parents will eat more healthily, they will begin to see benefits from doing so and ultimately will be protected from the chronic illnesses of later life to which obesity has been strongly connected as a risk factor. For want of a better word, she might think of all these things as producing more 'happiness' (or at least less misery).

But as Julie considers the possible beneficial consequences of the work, she also starts to recognise that its consequences might not be completely of benefit. In the same way that, according to some forms of utilitarianism, for an action to be viewed as moral it need only produce good effects (regardless of intentions), an action performed with good intentions and resulting in bad effects would be seen as unethical.

> Q. Can you think of any adverse or unintended consequences that might emerge from the healthy eating intervention? Make a note of these.

One possible adverse and unintended consequence might be that the intervention raises anxiety among some of those it is aimed at. Delivering lifestyle interventions not only carries potential good news ('You face this risk factor but you can do something about it'), but also potential bad news ('Carry on like this and you stand the chance of facing major illness'). While Julie and her colleagues undoubtedly intend to translate the potential good news into the *actually* positive, they cannot dismiss the possibility that anxieties will emerge. This might especially be the case if it appears that the change required to avoid later health problems is going to be just too difficult to achieve (Duncan and Cribb, 1996; Marteau, 1989, 1990).

Of course, awareness of this as a possible but unintended consequence of the intervention will help to shape it so that what is not intended can be avoided, or the chances of it happening might be minimised. But Julie is led on from the idea of this particular unintended consequence to consider that this intervention might give rise to multiple consequences, some of which may be difficult or impossible to foresee, or to do very much about. Children arguing with parents, school or practice staff suffering from stress because of the extra workload, youngsters rushing off to eat takeaway burgers in the face of 'health evangelists', and so on. The list of adverse consequences could be very long indeed.

Some consequentialist thinkers have recognised the difficulty within the idea that we cannot ever fully know all the possible effects of our actions. This has led to a distinction between two different kinds of utilitarianism. **Act** (or **extreme**) **utilitarians** hold that what we should do is to weigh up on *each occasion* when we are contemplating action which course will produce the greatest good (Smart, 1967). **Rule** (or **restricted**) **utilitarians** argue that what we should do is to obey action-guiding rules that we know, if they are generally followed, will result in the greatest good. But even this distinction does not quite deal with the problem of multiple and unforeseen consequences. If Julie decided to follow act utilitarianism, she would have the benefit of assessing the healthy eating intervention as an individual act, being undertaken in particular and unique circumstances. (There is nowhere quite like this, and no other set of children, parents, teachers and health care workers will be quite like this one.) However, this will not prevent unforeseen and adverse consequences occurring. Equally, if she were to apply rule utilitarianism, there is no guarantee that she would receive adequate guidance from the rules received. We might know generally that if we act in an inclusive way, if we use all available evidence, if we treat children and parents as individuals, if we work *with* rather than *for* people, good results follow. There is, though, no cast-iron guarantee of this, simply because the intervention has never been tried out in exactly these circumstances before.

The problem of multiple, possibly unforeseen and adverse consequences gets even more difficult if we return to thinking about what kind of outcomes, generally speaking, we are looking for. The utilitarian believes that we should aim to produce the greatest happiness for the greatest number. While Julie recognises that this might be one possible and quite reasonable goal for health services, she wonders whether it should be the only or the overriding one. We might argue, say, that an important goal of health services is fair distribution of scarce resources (Cribb, 2005). Undertaking actions that produce fair resource distribution as a consequence might directly conflict with the likelihood of 'greatest happiness' as an outcome. For example, fair distribution in the context of the healthy eating intervention might require that we concentrate on the small numbers of disadvantaged children and parents, and leave the affluent majority alone. This might be acceptable, but there is also a good chance that it might cause quite a few middle-class families some anguish.

Thinking About....

I have argued for at least two potential difficulties with a consequentialist (particularly utilitarian) approach to thinking about the healthy eating intervention. First, we cannot be sure that the intervention will only have the outcome intended. Second, even if the intended outcome (greatest happiness for the greatest number) is achieved, why should *this* be our moral priority?

Reflect on this assessment of a utilitarian approach to the intervention.

Conclusion: Obligations, Consequences and the Need for Action

At this point, Julie Seale admits to herself that she is perplexed! She has spent much time thinking about the healthy eating intervention through the lenses of deontological and consequentialist theories. She has debated it in her university class and is in the middle of writing an assignment about it. But so far she has come to no firm (or at least no positive) conclusion. The problem with a reliance on obligations (duties) is broadly that while they might be generally appropriate and applicable, they may not always be so under every circumstance. And the difficulty with allowing a concern for consequences to frame action is that they may be slippery, hard to identify and ultimately disputed.

Yet even at this stage of confusion, Julie recognises two things. First, thoughts about obligations and about consequences remain important components of any attempt at ethical thinking. She is now very aware of the difficulties with both deontology and consequentialism, but equally she knows that they can't be discounted. Reference to her ordinary everyday personal and professional experience tells her that in deciding how to act in the best (the most ethical) way, we think about both what we must do and what it would be best to do. These seem to her to be everyday shorthand for the idea that the vast majority of people have obligations or duties, and most of us have an awareness of the consequences of our actions.

The second thing Julie recognises is that there is a *need to act*. The healthy eating intervention won't go away. She is required to involve herself with it. Dr Williams is not going to change her mind. Even if she did, there would still be a need for some other kind of action. We have already discussed the huge public health importance of the problem of childhood obesity. If it is not work with schools and parents, some other initiative will be planned. It might even be implemented from on high through policy, or directives to practice. In Julie's view, it is better to act, and act with thoughtfulness, than not to act and have action forced upon you. The question, then, is whether there is a way of understanding obligations, consequences and values in the health care context that makes sense of conflicting demands and the messy experience of health care workers. This is the question that I will begin to address in the next chapter.

Chapter Summary

In this chapter, I have:

- Explored the nature of an obligation (or duty)-based theory of ethics;
- Explored the nature of a consequences-based theory of ethics;
- Considered both the possibilities and the problems attached to each of these kinds of theories when applied to the practical health care context.

Further Reading

Cottingham, J (ed.) (2008). *Western Philosophy: An Anthology*. Oxford: Blackwell. Writers such as Kant and Mill can be hard to get to grips with, but Cottingham's anthology provides bite-sized chunks of the philosophical classics, along with a helpful commentary.

Mackie, JL (1977). *Ethics: Inventing Right and Wrong*. Harmondsworth: Penguin. This is a good, although not an easy, introduction to ethical theory.

5

ETHICAL THINKING: THE FOUR PRINCIPLES OF HEALTH CARE ETHICS

Learning Outcomes

By the end of this chapter, you should be able to:

○ Describe and discuss the central claims made by some health care ethicists on behalf of the 'famous four' principles of health care ethics;
○ Describe and discuss the principles themselves;
○ Identify and discuss both possibilities and problems emerging from the principles and their application in the practical health care context.

Introduction

I spent some time in Chapter 3 discussing the renewed interest, from about the middle of the twentieth century, in the ethics of health care. The increasing technological capacity of medicine especially, and the distance it appeared to help create between health care workers and their patients, led to crises of public doubt and mistrust in those who were supposedly working for public benefit. One response to these crises was for those involved in health care to seek the help of professional ethicists – in the beginning mainly philosophers and theologians – and their experience of thinking about questions of values and moral purpose. In this way, what I have called 'bioethics' began to assume a more and more important place in the thinking of those engaged in health care.

What health care often appeared to be seeking from ethics was answers to questions of trust and direction in professional practice. It needed 'solutions' to urgent practical dilemmas; or at least it needed to show that it was responding to growing public concern about what it was doing (Jonsen, 1998). Given that it was mostly philosophers and theologians who were assuming the new mantle of 'bioethicist' and providing this response, it was natural that they should use their 'home' disciplines to supply the material from which they built up the occupation of bioethics.

One way or another, both philosophy and theology are concerned with values and what is valuable. I have already described and discussed the contrasting philosophical ethical projects of deontology and consequentialism. Each is concerned with production of the valuable: the first arguing that this lies broadly in keeping to action-guiding duties and obligations; the second that it rests in consideration of the consequences of action. This was the material that philosophers were bringing to the new bioethics. (Although as I have explained, the twentieth century had seen an increasing belief that these sorts of normative theories of ethics were misplaced or even misguided.)

Theology, too, had a concern with normative ethics. We can understand theology as the study of God, His dealings with humans and what it might mean to be human in a world He has created (Jonsen, 1998: 35). Given this, it is natural that the theologians who came to bioethics did so with normative conceptions of ethics that centred on the existence of a deity. For example, the noted theologian Paul Ramsey argues for deontological ethics because we have a duty of obedience in the light of God's overwhelming love for us (Ramsey, cited in Jonsen, 1998: 51).

Despite the difference in orientation of theologians and secular philosophers (one group bound to God and the other not), both were concerned to apply their traditions to understanding the moral problems of health care and the crisis in trust that it faced in the middle of the twentieth century. The fact that there were multiple traditions (both within and between those involved in the separate disciplines) that needed accounting for led to some people believing that what was required was a 'theory' of bioethics that could be widely accepted. We might call this approach **pluralist** (Jackson, 2006: 3).

Wide acceptance was required on the part of the bioethicists involved in theory construction and on the part of those they were aiming to help. One of the most 'successful' pluralist approaches to health care ethics is the so-called four principles approach, originally developed by two US bioethicists, Tom Beauchamp and James Childress (Beauchamp and Childress, 2001). The principles have been widely disseminated, at least through the English-speaking world, their cause being taken up enthusiastically in the UK by the general practitioner and ethicist Raanan Gillon (Gillon, 1990).

With this background in mind, my plan in this chapter is to describe and discuss the four principles framework. I want to examine the principles themselves and how they might be applied in the health care context (as well as the difficulties that might be connected to their application). But I also want to consider the claims made on their behalf by those who support the principles. Do they deserve their widespread dissemination? In their attempt at pluralism, is it the case that they really are generally acceptable to those working in health care (and by implication to the people whom health care workers serve)?

Introducing (or Re-introducing) the Four Principles of Health Care Ethics

In an article in the *British Medical Journal*, Raanan Gillon provides a summary of the four principles approach, beginning with an account of why he believes them to be important:

> The 'four principles plus scope' approach provides a simple, accessible and cultur-ally neutral approach to thinking about ethical issues in health care. The approach ... is based on four common, basic *prima facie* moral commitments – respect for autonomy, beneficence [the production of benefit], non-maleficence [the avoidance of harm], and justice – plus concern for their scope of application. It offers a com-mon, basic moral analytical framework and a common, basic moral language. (Gillon, 1994: 184)

I will consider what Gillon might mean by the '*prima facie*' nature of the principles and their 'scope of application' shortly, when I think more generally about the claims that are being made on their behalf. For the moment, a short introduction to the principles themselves is needed. For some, this may indeed be a re-introduction as they have been very effectively promulgated in many health care teaching and learning contexts.

The principle of respect for autonomy

Autonomy is our capacity to engage in 'deliberated self-rule' (Gillon, 1994: 185). In other words, it is possessing control over our own lives and their direction. There are different kinds (or levels) of autonomy. **Autonomy of thought** is the capacity to think and reason, hold moral views, political preferences, and so on. We can understand **autonomy of will** as the ability to intend to perform an action as a result of thought and reason. **Autonomy of action** is the capacity freely to act in accordance with the intentions that someone has developed. We can restrict our own autonomy (or have it restricted for us) at any of these lev-els. For example, Ian is a nurse who is actively involved in his trades union. The local union decides that there should be a work to rule to protest against what is seen as management victimisation of another member of staff. Ian agrees with the work to rule (autonomy of thought) and speaks in favour of it at his local branch meeting (autonomy of will). However, when he next turns up for a shift, he is faced with a ward full of dependent patients. One of the important elements of the work to rule is taking the full time allowed for breaks. Ian now has a dilemma. Does he do this (comply with the work to rule) and leave this demanding ward short-staffed for a while? Or does he carry on with his usual practice of either not taking a break or taking a shorter one than he is allowed (break the work to rule)? It doesn't matter what he eventually does – the point is that there are actual or potential restrictions on his autonomy of action.

The **principle of respect for autonomy** is the moral obligation we may believe we have to respect the autonomy of others, to the extent that this respect is compatible with the autonomy of all those actually or potentially affected by the action being considered. That is to say, we are free to act so long as our actions do not adversely affect the autonomy of others. I am free to study far into the night for my ethics and health care course. I am not free to study far into the night while at the same time playing loud music because this would affect the autonomy of my neighbours (their freedom to sleep without disturbance).

The principle of beneficence

This is the moral commitment we might believe we have to **produce benefit** for those we serve. Most usually, health care professionals understand this commitment as being towards their patients or clients. The principle of beneficence cannot be considered alone, but must always be part of an assessment also involving the next principle, that of non-maleficence (avoidance of harm).

The principle of non-maleficence

The moral obligation that we may believe we hold to **avoid harm** is inevitably closely connected to the principle of beneficence. Any intervention or action carries at least the *potential* risk that it will result in harm as well as produce benefit. In order for a health care intervention to be considered 'ethical', it must always produce net benefit over harm (Gillon, 1994: 185). This assessment of 'benefit divided by harm' is often a very difficult one to undertake but, as we have already seen, we cannot assume that any health care action, no matter how well intentioned, will automatically result in good, or benefit. (Consider again the example of Julie Seale and the healthy eating intervention, in which she thought hard about the anxieties and tensions for parents and children that could emerge from the actions she was involved in planning.)

The principle of concern for justice

The principle of concern for justice is the obligation we may believe we have to act on the basis of **fair adjudication between competing claims related to health care**. The resources available for health care will always be scarce, even in affluent Western societies (Palmer and Ho, 2008). Thus, one element of a concern for justice is to make sure that resources are distributed fairly (**distributive justice**). Another aspect of health care-related justice is what might be called **natural rights**. As human beings, we expect to be treated with dignity, to have our wishes and preferences at least considered, if not acted on, to live as far as possible without fear of pain and physical or mental abuse. Ensuring that these sorts of rights are maintained and any attempt to challenge them is obstructed is the territory of **rights-based justice**. Finally, we expect that health care professionals will follow the law and that we will receive our legal entitlements with regard to care (**legal justice**). This latter aspect of concern for justice is rather problematic, however, for courts and judges have traditionally been reluctant to make judgements about what are legal entitlements in specific cases of treatment and care (Duncan, 2008).

'Subsidiary' principles

One criticism sometimes made of the principles is that they are so broad as to be vacuous (Hare, 1994). If we talk about an obligation to 'produce benefit', for example, what exactly do we mean? I will consider more specific aspects of this criticism shortly, but for the time being it's important to note that key supporters of the principles, such as Gillon, seem to view them as being at the apex of a more content-filled triangle. Beneath the principle of beneficence, for example, would be what we might call 'subsidiary' principles. These would support the broad principle of the production of benefit. Subsidiary principles connected to beneficence might include things like the commitment to research (so that we know what is effective and what works), the commitment to ongoing continuing professional development, and so on. In this way, the importance of the broad principle remains, but it assumes more content through the subsidiary principles that flow from it.

Thinking About...

I have sketched out some of the subsidiary principles that might emerge as a result of a commitment to the principle of beneficence. Reflect on what form they might take for the remaining principles (respect for autonomy, non-maleficence and concern for justice).

The Importance of the Four Principles: Claims from Bioethics

Now I want to unpack the claims that have been made for the four principles approach in a little more detail and in doing so start to develop a critique of it. Supporters of the principles and the approach they represent are not shy of making claims for them, and for their use to those working in health care and thinking about its problems. Jennifer Jackson offers the following interpretation of Beauchamp and Childress's (and by association Gillon's) position. Whether or not it is possible to construct a comprehensive ethical theory does not matter:

> At least, it does not matter for the project of practical ethics. All the rival theories, they [Beauchamp and Childress] say, converge in agreement with the four principles that can provide the basis and framework for biomedical ethics. (Jackson, 2006: 3)

Jackson's representation of this claim (which she does not necessarily agree with) suggests the following. The attempts at comprehensive ethical theory that we discussed in the previous chapter (deontology and consequentialism) are problematic on their own, but they can be reconciled and united under the banner of the four principles. This is because:

- The principles are sufficiently wide to be accepted as reasonable values that those in health care should be trying to defend and develop (and so as a framework they contain an important consequentialist component);
- They are nevertheless framed as commitments or obligations that are applicable in the vast majority of health care situations, and which we need to try to follow (therefore they can also be seen as having a deontological component).

This moves us towards examining the key claims of acceptability and applicability that are made for the four principles approach.

Acceptability and applicability

In the first place, the principles, their supporters claim, are (or should be) widely acceptable. Regardless of our occupational or professional background and training, our culture, religion or politics, we should be able to commit to them. This in itself is a large claim, for two reasons:

- We live and work in a diverse, multicultural society, containing a wide variety of political and religious beliefs, or non-beliefs. This is an empirical fact (Douglas et al., 2007). Given this, the search for values that we can all subscribe to is difficult (Bogdanor et al., 2007). Some believe in social co-operation, others in individualism. Some believe in supporting people as necessary in the development of their social capital, others that it is individuals' own responsibility to make their way in the world and it's too bad for those who are not able to do so (Neuberger, 2005). Against this backdrop, can the four principles approach really represent the values that we ought to hold with regard to health care?
- I spent some time in Chapter 2 describing the process by which health care workers might acquire the values they hold. I argued that this process was, in itself, a good part of the reason why the values held by those working in health care are so firmly embedded. The question now is whether we can agree that the four principles are sufficiently representative of the values that are already strongly present in health care and its occupations.

In the second place, those defending the principles argue that they are applicable to most ethical situations in health care. This again is a substantial claim. An argument of this book so far has been that ethics is of wide and crucial relevance to anyone working in health care, at any time of his or her practice. Given what we know about the breadth of health care activity and interest (think again of Dr Irwin and Mrs Murphy, Joe the autistic boy and Julie Seale with her involvement in healthy eating), this suggests very wide relevance. But wide *relevance* is not the same as wide *applicability*. I can argue that ethical questions appear in all aspects of health care, but this is different from suggesting that there is a framework for understanding and responding to them that we can apply to every context and situation.

If we are to treat the four principles seriously, and properly assess how useful they might be to us in our own search for frameworks that enable understanding and debate, at least part of our evaluation of them needs to centre on these questions:

- Are they *really* widely acceptable in our multicultural society?
- Are they *really* applicable to most moral situations in health care?

Thinking About...

Consider whether you believe it is possible for a set of ethical principles to be widely applicable and acceptable, given the plurality of our society and the broad nature of health care work.

I will return to these questions later in the chapter. For the time being, I want to consider some further claims made in relation to the four principles.

The principles as *prima facie*

Gillon talks of the principles as 'four common, basic *prima facie* moral commitments' (Gillon, 1994: 184). What exactly does '*prima facie*' mean? The dictionary defines it as:

> At first sight, based on a first impression. ... One that seemed, at first sight, to be valid. (Oxford University Press, 1983)

There is a slightly different, but complementary, philosophical understanding of the term, from the moral philosopher WD Ross, who understood that a *prima facie* principle is one that is binding, unless it conflicts with another principle. In other words, when we approach a moral issue in health care, our responsibility in the first place is to consider it against the four principles of respect for autonomy, beneficence, non-maleficence and justice. If we are in doubt about how to act, we need to assess the situation and consider how best any action that we undertake would meet the demands of the principles. Would it respect autonomy? How? Would it support the exercise of justice in the health care context? And so on. We must follow the principles unless there is conflict between them. Supporters of the principles readily admit that there will be cases where there is such conflict – say, between my desire to respect a patient's autonomy and a concern for the exercise of justice.

Example

Dr Irwin is respecting Mrs Murphy's autonomy because she wishes to die. However, his actions in support of her suicide militate against the principle of justice (at least legal justice) because it is presently against the law to assist someone in the taking of their own life. So in this example there is conflict between at least two of the *prima facie* principles.

An easy objection to the four principles approach lies in this idea of conflict between the principles. What use are they if they do not provide definitive guidance? The objection is easy, but it is important. Health care professionals are busy people, often working in pressured circumstances, so they might well be entitled to think that an expectation of guidance is quite reasonable.

A defence against this objection would argue that any claim for the principles to be prescriptively action-guiding mistakes their purpose. Here, the context within which they have been developed becomes important. We live in a pluralist society so what we require is not prescriptive rules but instead: 'A common set of moral commitments, a common moral language, and a common set of moral issues' (Gillon, 1994: 184). We know that we will encounter a wide range of contexts involving different people with variations in beliefs and values. So what is needed is some common ground for discussion. Let's consider the following analogy. My family can't agree where we will spend the Christmas holiday next year. There are a number of possibilities. We could spend it at home. We could go and stay with one or other of our extended family. We could go away to a luxurious hotel. Or we could volunteer to help at the local day centre where lunch will be served for older people who might otherwise be on their own. There would probably be no point in me trying to *prescribe* what everyone should do ('We're all going to stay with Cousin Annie'), not least because my family would start digging their heels in at the thought ('But her house is always so cold and she feeds her dogs from the table'). But what *would* probably be helpful is to set down a number of principles that we might broadly be able to agree on and according to which we might choose what to do – or at least that would help us to make the choice. These could include, for example, the requirement not to travel very far, the need not to spend too much money, and the need for us not to feel totally selfish and have some purpose in the use of our time. This might lead us to decline the offer from Cousin Annie, say, and think seriously about the day centre instead.

What we have done here is to establish a way in which we might talk about our Christmas holiday options without losing our tempers or setting our face against possibilities. Equally, with regard to the four principles, we are not defining or prescribing action, but rather establishing a common ground, which will enable us to debate potential choices and through the process of debate become clearer about what is at stake (and ultimately what we might do).

The principles and their scope of application

The four principles approach, Gillon writes, is based on the principles themselves, plus a concern for their 'scope of application'. His argument at this point is that while we may agree we hold obligations to respect autonomy, produce benefit, avoid harm and have concern for justice, it cannot be said (necessarily) that we hold these obligations towards everyone. So there is a need to think carefully about exactly *to whom* we do in fact owe these obligations.

Q. To whom do you think health care workers (or those training to work in health care) owe moral obligations?

Gillon argues that in general terms health care workers owe the obligations set out in the four principles approach to their patients or clients. This is because those working as professionals in health care, by virtue of making their 'profession', have offered a commitment to help patients or clients, to do them no harm, and so on. This commitment is enshrined and embedded in various ways, through institutional and organisational rules, legal frameworks, professional codes of conduct, etc. However, it is too easy and unreflective to say that we owe all the obligations contained in the principles to all of our patients or clients all of the time.

Think back to the three cases in Chapter 1. In respecting Mrs Murphy's autonomy, Dr Irwin was arguably stepping beyond normal expectations with regard to autonomy respect because he was allowing her to carry through the autonomous decision to commit suicide. In doing so, he was probably breaking the law as it stands. We can understand this as a conflict between a general principle and a specific regulation, which places possible limits on autonomy respect. Even so, we can still argue about what should be done. Equally, the case of childhood obesity poses a dilemma. Should we respect the autonomy of people to have the kind of diet they want, regardless of the possible health effects? And if we do, can we also hold that we should respect the autonomy of people who, having spent 20 or 30 years eating whatever they want, now require us to agree that they should have expensive surgery or other treatment? We can see this also as a question of possibly limiting autonomy in particular cases. Finally, the case of Joe, the severely autistic boy, also raises questions of limits to autonomy, even in the context of the professional–patient relationship. Say, for example, that Joe enters hospital for a short period of treatment. While there, he (seemingly deliberately and knowingly) puts himself in harm's way. Should those caring for him stop this from happening? We might believe that we are more entitled to do so with Joe than with somebody who is not severely autistic. But what are our grounds for this belief? Thinking about the principle of respect for autonomy in relation to Joe's situation again suggests that we may not owe this obligation to patients or clients all of the time.

One of the things that is clear in this consideration of the principles' scope of application is that much depends on who we are talking about, and the context in which they live. Our reactions to questions about the extent to which people should exercise autonomy with regard to choosing death, ill-health and harm (among other things) are not simply determined by the fact that the people concerned are our patients or clients. For example, our thoughts about the degree to which Mrs Murphy is 'allowed' to decide on her death are strongly shaped by the fact that we know she is suffering from severe pain and at the end stages of terminal illness. We might agree that in general we hold the obligations contained in the principles to our patients or clients, but not always. This is an important point, for two reasons:

- It does not prejudice the principles themselves; it simply raises questions about their scope of application (I am not challenging, say, the principle of respect for autonomy in itself, but I might question whether it applies in a particular situation) (Gillon, 1994: 187);
- This recognition ought to commit us to an ever-present reflective concern for scope.

In this way, the principles, at least according to a supporter like Gillon, fulfil their promise of providing a common moral language through which we can debate particular issues. Going back to my earlier non-health example, my family can't have a debate about where we will be going next Christmas holiday unless we are able to agree on what we might be seeking generally from this time off. Analogously, we can't debate specific situations in health care unless we have a general idea of what our moral commitments in the field might be. We now need to return to the questions we raised before: Can we agree that the principles are *generally* acceptable? Can we agree on their *general* applicability?

Evaluating the Principles: Claims and Content

In order to evaluate the four principles approach and the claims made on its behalf, my plan is to consider their use in the context of three different kinds of example. Each example has been chosen to highlight one kind of evaluative problem with the approach, although I also want to argue that there is overlap between the problems. Issues of applicability, say, also affect questions of acceptability and *vice versa*. However, it is possible to imagine at least one counter-argument to my own approach.

An argument against my own way of evaluating the four principles, through the use of a small number of hypothetical examples, is to say that I have been highly selective in my choice of scenarios. I have deliberately tailored them to draw out problems. This is certainly true (after all, I have a case to make!), but in defence I would want to claim the following:

- These are not extraordinary examples. They could form part of the everyday practice or concern of many health care professionals – what I have tended to call 'ordinary' health care. If these examples might form part of ordinary practice, and if they demonstrate problems with the principles, then it could be the case that those problems are widespread in practice itself, well beyond my examples.
- These examples are not being used with the intention of trying to demolish the principles. Their widespread use suggests that they are helpful to many engaged in health care and this is the conclusion that I will eventually reach. However, before it is possible to do so, if we are being properly analytic and reflective in our approach, we need to consider potential difficulties.

Thinking About...

Read through the examples I have provided below and consider whether or not they do (as I claim) represent everyday practice and concern.

Applicability: conflict between the principles

Example

Jonathan Barker is an occupational therapist working for a local NHS Health Care Trust. He is involved in arranging for the discharge from hospital of Mrs Elizabeth Lucas, an 82 year-old widow who has suffered a number of falls at home and was finally admitted six weeks ago with an acute chest infection. As part of the discharge procedure, Jonathan organises a home visit to the part-warden-controlled flat where she lives alone.

Mrs Lucas is adamant that she wants to return home. She does not want to enter residential care, the only other option available. However, the home visit goes very badly, with Mrs Lucas unable to perform essential tasks of daily living. Finally, she breaks down in tears, pleading to be allowed to stay in her own home.

Jonathan knows that the most practical option would be for Mrs Lucas to enter a situation where more care would be immediately available to her. Yet it is quite clear that she does not want to do this. Anything other than remaining in the flat is unacceptable to her.

The issue of applicability here relates to conflict between the principles. Should the overriding commitment be towards respecting Mrs Lucas's autonomy and doing everything possible to ensure that she stays in her flat? Or should the commitment be towards another principle or principles? Jonathan knows that there is substantial risk of harm occurring and benefit not being produced if Mrs Lucas stays where she is. (She is very likely to fall again and her levels of self-care may well deteriorate.) Non-maleficence and beneficence seem quite reasonable moral commitments to Jonathan in this case, to the extent that they might possibly trump the principle of respect for autonomy. But how is he to choose what to recommend to the case conference that will follow the visit? Should he be recommending anything at all?

I have already briefly discussed in general terms the potential problem of conflict between the principles. Through this example, though, what I am doing is to consider it in relation to claims for the widespread applicability of the principles. My original defence against principles conflict was that while they didn't provide definitive answers, they could contribute towards a common moral language to enable discussion (Gillon, 1994: 184). But the problem in the example of Mrs Lucas is that, as Jonathan faces the case conference, there seems to be the possibility that he needs to engage with two separate kinds of language. One is the language of empowerment and self-direction embedded within the principle of respect for autonomy. The other is the language of professional expertise and risk assessment embodied by the principles of non-malefience and beneficence as they might apply to Mrs Lucas's case. In terms of discussion about the applicability of the principles, the central question is this: Can we properly regard them as generally applicable when they generate quite different ways of seeing the purpose and nature of health care? The breadth of the commitments proposed by the principles suggests the real possibility of conflict not only between them, but also between the separate paradigms of understanding and care that they seem to represent. It is one thing to debate between principles. It is quite another, and much more difficult, to debate between separate paradigms.

Applicability: the problem of knowledge

Example

Karen Locke is a staff nurse on a busy surgical ward. She has been asked to admit Derek Kingsley to her ward. Mr Kingsley is a 35 year-old computer programmer who is to undergo day surgery for the removal of a fibroma (believed to be benign) on his arm. While going through the admissions procedure, Karen discovers that Mr Kingsley's regular weekly alcohol consumption is the equivalent of 60 units per week. This is more than twice the limit recommended by the NHS of 3–4 units a day (that is, 21–28 units per week) for men (National Health Service/Home Office, 2008). Karen wonders whether she should offer strong advice to Mr Kingsley on the levels of his drinking.

The difficulty here is not so much one of framing a discussion about what should be done in the context of the principles, although, as with the previous example, we might well disagree about which course of action to choose. Karen could be motivated by the principle of beneficence and offer the advice in the hope that Mr Kingsley will act on it. In doing so, she would have to weigh up the possibility of raising alarm in Mr Kingsley about his health behaviour and in some practical way would have to 'square' beneficence with non-maleficence. It is relatively easy to imagine Karen having this kind of debate (perhaps with herself, possibly with colleagues) about what to do. But underlying this debate is a much more pervasive difficulty: if Karen were to intervene (or even if she did not), *what difference would it make*? In other words, do we know enough about the effects of alcohol consumption and of alcohol-related behaviour to say that if Mr Kingsley cut down on his drinking, his health would improve?

There are two things to say in response to this question. First, the recommended 'sensible drinking' limits decided on by the government (21–28 units for men and 14–21 units for women per week) are subject to dispute. Some have argued that they have been imposed more from a concern for social control than as a result of firm epidemiological evidence (Fitzpatrick, 2001). So while Karen might intuitively think that 60 units per week is 'too much' and advise cutting down to the recommended limits, the actual evidence that this will result in better health for Mr Kingsley is problematic. Second, there is a need to ask whether this kind of brief, opportunistic intervention would actually change Mr Kingsley's behaviour anyway? There is evidence to suggest that the effect of health promotion interventions on behaviour change is limited and that, in any case, for alteration to occur the intervention has to be more sustained and longer-lasting (Family Heart Study Group, 1994; Imperial Cancer Research Fund Oxcheck Study Group, 1995).

These difficulties with what we might call 'evidence of effectiveness' are widespread in the field of health promotion, although they are not confined only to this aspect of health care. Within 'mainstream' practice, there are different and conflicting views about the nature of evidence and what 'counts' in decision-making. The occasions when we are able to rely on the supposed 'gold standard' of health care research, the randomised controlled trial (RCT) to inform our practice are limited (Cribb and Duncan, 2002).

Thinking About...

The RCT is regarded as the 'gold standard' to which medical and health care research should aspire (Tones and Green, 2004). RCTs involve the random division of a given population into the 'experimental' group, which receives the treatment, procedure or intervention being tested, and the 'control' group, which does not. If the two groups are matched for characteristics, then any differences between the groups will be as a result of the intervention (Earle et al., 2007).

Consider and reflect on the extent to which your different daily practices in health care are actually based on this 'gold standard'.

The point in thinking about the 'gold standard' of the RCT is not to try to claim weakness in our daily practice. Instead, it is to assert that this practice is often difficult, messy and based on a mixture of intuition and pragmatism, and the requirements of organisations and policy. The extent to which 'strong' research evidence, such as that generated through RCTs, actually guides our practice is likely to be limited. In the example of Karen and Mr Kingsley, there is a short answer to the question, 'Do we know enough about the effects of alcohol consumption and of alcohol-related behaviour to say that if Mr Kingsley cut down on his drinking, his health would improve?' The answer is 'No'. This doesn't mean that Karen shouldn't offer advice (there are all kinds of reasons why she should). However, what it does mean in the context of the four principles approach is that the benefit over harm equation that the principles require us to work out in this kind of situation (and in lots of others) is likely to be very difficult. This is simply because of the problems associated with the health care 'evidence base' itself.

Acceptability: whose needs and wishes should count?

Example

Ayesha Khan works as a public health specialist in an East London borough. The borough has very high rates of social deprivation and a wide diversity of population. Minority ethnic communities account for close to 50% of the total borough population.

Ayesha is working with the local community relations council on a project that aims to provide sexual health information to a small section of the Bangladeshi community living in a particular part of the borough. The project has come about because a health needs assessment conducted recently, and involving a number of young women from the community, identified a gap in knowledge and understanding of issues such as contraception, HIV/AIDS and other sexually transmitted diseases.

At first glance, this seems like an unproblematic example. Work has been undertaken to identify a health need that is currently unmet, and the plan now is to address this need. The young women who supported the needs assessment are enthusiastic about the project. It certainly appears as if principles such as beneficence and respect for autonomy are being met. The difficulty, however, is that these young women are a small minority of the community. The larger community, in particular its male elders, take a very different view on the provision of sexual health information to women from the younger generation, regarding it as promoting promiscuity and infidelity. The question here is one of whose wishes and needs should count. Should it be those of the women themselves? Or should it be those of the broader community, as represented by its elders?

Whichever position Ayesha and her fellow workers take, the example draws attention to the fact that the principles are grounded in a particular moral and social tradition – what we might call 'Western liberalism'. There are some who would claim that this tradition gives rise to the idea that autonomy is the most fundamental value, to be promoted as diligently as possible by health care workers (Bowles et al., 2006). Thus the principle of respect for autonomy assumes the status of 'first among equals' (*primus intra pares*) within the four principles approach (Seedhouse, 1998). But in a pluralistic and multicultural society such as that in the United Kingdom, there is an important need to ask whether liberalism and, in particular, the principle of respect for autonomy can reasonably be argued to 'trump' all other potential positions based on different sorts of values. In this example, Ayesha is confronted in particular by the alternative values of paternalism (the male elders know best) and possibly communitarianism (the needs and wishes of the whole community are what counts and not those of a small minority of young women). Both of these values could deeply influence our interpretation of the principles' relevance in the context of the sexual health information project, and what might actually be done. For example, if we are guided by the value of paternalism, the principle of respect for autonomy becomes much less important (maybe even irrelevant). And the principle of beneficence might be interpreted as the production of benefit in so far as the paternalistic structures of the community Ayesha is working with are maintained and protected.

> Q:• What do you think is the most important value in this context, and therefore
> •the one that those concerned should try to promote through their interpretation and application of one or more of the four principles?

Whatever conclusion you have come to as a result of considering this question, perhaps the crucial point is that disagreement is possible. It is possible here (and in other similar examples) because either the principles themselves or our interpretation of them as health care workers might not be acceptable to those with whom we are working. In particular, the broadly liberal concerns of Western health care ethics (reflecting the liberal contexts of the Western societies from which it has emerged) might conflict with the different kinds of values present in some parts of our multicultural society (Buruma, 2007).

We need to add this analysis to those that I undertook in relation to the examples of Jonathan Barker and the home assessment, and Karen Locke and 'lifestyle advice'. Jonathan was confronted particularly with the problem of conflict between the principles (what Mrs Lucas wanted and what was 'best' for her). Karen faced the difficulty of uncertainty about the evidence that she might use to support her application of the principles. It's possible to summarise the problems we've encountered in applying the four principles approach to examples that might occur in practice in the following way:

- The applicability of the principles in at least some cases might be limited because of the conflict engendered between them;
- Their applicability might be lessened because on occasions (maybe even often) we are not sure of the evidence supporting a particular course of action that might be suggested by one or more of the principles;
- The emergence of the principles from the tradition of Western ethical liberalism might mean that they conflict with values (and consequent principles) important to at least some sections of our multicultural society.

Conclusion: 'Moral Strangers' and Practical Necessity

Much of the difficulty with the four principles approach lies in the fact that it has been constructed in uncertain times (Englehardt Jr and Wildes, 1994). As we have seen in this and previous chapters, there are at least three kinds of uncertainties that health care workers face that are likely to affect their capacity to apply the approach in their practice:

- Increasing uncertainty about the status and authority of the professional role (as a result of public mistrust born of health care 'scandals' and 'unstoppable technology') means that the question of whose views and values should count has become much more relevant. It is certainly no longer enough for the professional to say, 'I'm doing this for your benefit'. Professional thoughts about benefit and harm, for example, need to be much more carefully considered, given that patients or clients may well be very dubious about, or even actively challenging of, our position on such things.
- Increasing uncertainty and contest about the evidence that supports health care decision-making. The health care evidence base is constantly evolving and growing, but it is also subject to greater and greater questioning and challenge. In particular, the assumption that positivist enquiry and evidence gathered through the use of quantitative methodologies is what counts is being questioned by those committed to theories based around the idea that our knowledge and understanding is socially constructed (Broom and Willis, 2007). Given the requirement for evidence to support deliberation over the principles, dispute about the nature, reliability and ideology underpinning the health care evidence base cannot be helpful for their application.
- Increasing uncertainty about overarching social values. In a multicultural society, we cannot rely on everybody agreeing that the foundation of liberalism, which seems to underpin the four principles approach, is acceptable and uniformly valuable to all.

This has led some to argue that in the so-called postmodern era of shifting values and constantly altering relationships of power and influence, an attempt to pare health care ethics down to a set of principles is doomed to failure. It will fail because our postmodern condition does not allow us to have sufficient in common, morally speaking, with those who are around us. We are 'moral strangers' to each other:

> Moral strangers do not see the world in the same way. They do not possess common content-full moral premises so as to resolve concrete moral controversies or agree regarding the nature of true human flourishing. (Engelhardt Jr and Wildes, 1994: 136)

So debate using the principles as a framework is impossible because we could never agree it is these particular principles that count in the first place. The solution offered to the problem of the four principles in a world of 'moral strangers' is to place the single principle of autonomy (now recast as the principle of 'consent') as the only one that should guide health care actions. If we are all strangers to each other, then what is most important is that we ask permission for whatever action we seek to undertake (Engelhardt Jr and Wildes, 1994: 137).

One obvious difficulty with this principle of consent is that there are some (possibly many) occasions in health care where consent can not be given – at least not directly by the patient or client concerned. Think of some of the cases and examples that I have presented so far. Consider Joe, the severely autistic boy, whose cognitive capacity might limit consenting ability. Think about Julie

Seale and healthy eating – can she really be expected to gain consent from everybody who might ultimately be touched by this public health project? Consider Mrs Lucas, struggling to stay in her home – would her understandably very strong emotions allow her to think in careful, 'consenting' terms?

I will discuss the issue of consent in health care more fully in Chapter 7. For the time being, we can suggest that the principle of respect for autonomy framed here as the principle of permission or consent is clearly very important (perhaps overriding). However, it does not seem to be able to account for *all* that we would want to say about ethical action in health care. There are occasions when assessment of benefit and harm are important, or where wider considerations, such as those related to justice, apply. Moreover, there is a practical necessity that we consider such questions in order to reach reasonable decisions about what to do. Arguing that gaining consent is the *only thing* that matters is not the same as arguing that it is a highly important component of ethical action. While we cannot ignore, and have to think carefully about, the substantial difficulties within an approach to ethics based on the four principles, their function in providing a framework for debate has to be taken seriously. So too does our capacity to engage in ethical thinking, and to understand the ground from which we work. This is the focus of the next chapter.

Chapter Summary

In this chapter, I have:

- Described and discussed the background to the four principles approach within health care ethics;
- Described and discussed the four principles themselves, together with related concepts;
- Discussed some of the difficulties connected to the approach, especially those related to their applicability and their acceptability, given the nature of health care and the social context in which it is practised.

Further Reading

Beauchamp, TL and JF Childress (2001). *Principles of Biomedical Ethics* (Fifth Edition). New York: Oxford University Press. This is the book in which Beuchamp and Childress first laid out the four principles approach. Many regard it as the most influential text on bioethics that has been written.

Gillon, R and A Lloyd (eds) (1994). *Principles of Health Care Ethics*. Chichester: Wiley This is an edited collection containing chapters by a number of authors that support, reflect on or critique the four principles approach.

6

ETHICS FROM THE 'OUTSIDE IN' OR THE 'INSIDE OUT'? CODES OF CONDUCT AND 'VIRTUOUS LIVES'

Learning Outcomes

By the end of this chapter, you should be able to:

○ Describe and discuss the purpose and nature of codes of conduct for health care professionals;
○ Discuss potential weaknesses within a codes-based approach to dealing with ethical difficulties in the health care context;
○ Describe and critically discuss the idea of 'learned virtue' as a counterpoint to the codes-based approach;
○ Describe and discuss the relationship between codes and virtues.

Introduction

Much of my concern so far has been to become clear about the nature of values in health care, and how normative systems of ethics (in particular deontology and consequentialism) might be applied to preserve or increase these values. What I have not spent much time doing so far is to explore how we might *develop* our understanding of what we should do, in an ethical sense, and why we should do it. The purpose of this chapter is to start that exploration, which will continue one way or another for much of the rest of the book.

Perhaps this seems an unnecessary project. 'Why do you need to do this?' someone might ask. Surely, it's enough that you've established what values are, what kinds of values might be important in the health care context and how philosophers and others have thought – or might think – about how action could be justified. We can either agree or otherwise with what you, and the philosophers whose ethical thinking you have been discussing, have actually said. Nothing more is needed. So long as we have enough of an understanding of ethical positions and systems, that will be sufficient to get us by. Trying to develop an understanding of how and why we do what we do is just going to complicate things. When I drive a car, I know there are certain things that I should and shouldn't do – techniques for driving, rules of the road, and so on. What's the point in me spending a lot of time thinking about how I've developed that understanding, and why I should obey the Highway Code? Either I do, or I get stopped by the police.

> Q. Do you agree with this assertion or not? Whether or not you agree, list your reasons for the position that you have taken.

It seems to me that there are at least three reasons why we should be doubtful about this assertion:

- It demonstrates a rather unreflective position. Continuing with the driving analogy, it is certainly true that we can spend a lifetime driving without thinking about how we've developed our understanding of the skill and its practice, or why we need to do what we do. At the same time, though, our lack of reflection means that we are hampered in becoming better drivers. We simply do what we have to. This may be enough, but what if the rules change? What if there is a requirement that our knowledge and understanding is reassessed (through periodic driving re-tests, say)? In both cases, if we have thought about how we do what we do, and why we do it, we will be better equipped to cope with the new situation.
- The driving analogy is *only* an analogy. In the case of unreflective obedience to the Highway Code, it's unlikely that this will lead us into too much trouble. In fact, it's possible that it will actually keep us out of trouble. Always asking why I should obey this red light in this circumstance (a seemingly deserted road, no other traffic) may well be a recipe for disaster. But health care ethics isn't exactly like this. Certainly, there will be some situations where it is quite clear what we should do (situations encompassed by the law, for example). But there will also be many circumstances where what we should do isn't clear at all. In these sorts of situations, knowing how we've developed our understanding (and can continue to develop it) as well as why we make the moral choices that we do is crucially important. Otherwise, we will simply be meeting uncertainty with confusion.
- In Chapter 2, I spent some time discussing the idea that the values held by health care workers are deeply embedded by virtue of their inculcation through long periods of professional training and their sustenance through professional lives (Duncan, 2007). I want to suggest again that we therefore need to be very careful in our examination of these values (and the positions they might lead to), how we've developed them and why we hold them. If we are not, we risk being slaves to the values that have been inculcated within us.

In this chapter, then, I am going to explore two alternative and apparently contrasting ways of understanding how we might develop our ethical thinking, and why we must act in particular fashions. The first is what I will call an 'outside in' way. By this I mean that we receive our ethical thinking and justification for action from outside sources. Here, those outside sources are understood as professional codes of conduct (but they could comprise other things, such as received religious or political beliefs, and so on). The second is an 'inside out' way. By this I mean that our thinking and justification for action come somehow from within us. (I borrow this 'outside in' and 'inside out' distinction from Angus Dawson (1994).) My focus in this chapter is on so-called virtue theory as a way of understanding how and why we might develop our moral capacity, but 'inside out' thinking might also include traditions such as Intuitionism. This is the idea that our intuitions play a central part in our deciding to act as we do, and that understanding and theorising these is an important philosophical project (Audi, 2004).

In other words, codes of conduct on the one hand, and virtue theory on the other, will be treated as *representatives* of the two apparently contrasting traditions of ethics from the 'outside in' and ethics from the 'inside out'. This will help sharpen our focus on the differences between the two but, as I will later argue, there is also a need to understand how and why there might be a relationship between them. I hope you are beginning to sense by now that ethics and its application to health care is often very resistant towards attempts at sharp focus and clear divisions!

Ethics from the 'Outside In': Codes of Conduct and their Purpose

If you belong to, or are training to join, a health care-related profession, there is a high likelihood that it will possess its own code of conduct or professional guidelines (see, for example, British Association of Social Workers, 2002; College of Occupational Therapy, 2001; Nursing and Midwifery Council, 2004).

Thinking About...

Find and review the code of conduct (it may be called code of ethics or professional guidelines) for your own profession, or the profession you are training to enter. If you are not currently a member of a profession or in professional training, review one of the documents that I have provided references for above. Reflect on what the *purpose* of the code that you have reviewed might be.

In the broadest sense, the purpose of codes of conduct is to guide professional practice. However, I want to argue that practice guidance is only one of the purposes of codes. Moreover, this particular purpose and its impact can only be properly understood through recognition and awareness of their other purposes.

Codes of conduct (while these kinds of documents are sometimes referred to by other names, such as codes of practice, I will use this term throughout my discussion) have both **internal** and **external purpose**. By 'internal', I mean that they serve to benefit the profession concerned and so, of course, its members. By 'external', I mean that they exist to convey something about the profession to the wider public and especially those who might be seeking the profession's particular services. They have, if you like, 'public relations' purposes. (Of course, internal and external purposes are linked; if a profession is perceived as having good relations with its public, this can only be of benefit to the members of the profession itself.) So as well as trying to provide guidance for professional practice (an internal purpose), codes have the following external purposes:

- They declare professional intent to their public. ('If you have cause to seek the services of nursing [or social work or whatever], we will attempt to serve you as well as we can.')
- They guarantee standards. ('Our attempt to serve you well will be underpinned by very specific commitments.')

These external purposes lead in turn to a further internal purpose:

- Through declaration of intent and guarantee of standards, codes bind a profession together. They assert a common unity in what the profession is about and how it achieves its social function (Edgar, 1994).

Crucially, although I argue that these are the purposes of codes of conduct, they cannot be achieved just by the code itself. Take, for example, the Nursing and Midwifery Council Code (Nursing and Midwifery Council (NMC), 2004). This follows what is the usual sort of format for such documents. It begins with a broad declaration of what the Council expects from members of the profession of nursing. It moves from these broad declarations to more specific expectations related to the declarations. So, for example, one of the broad declarations is:

> As a registered nurse, midwife or specialist community public health nurse, you are personally accountable for your practice. In caring for patients and clients, you must:
>
> Respect the patient or client as an individual. (NMC, 2004: 3)

In relation to this, the practitioner must:

> Recognise and respect the role of patients and clients as partners in their care and the contribution they can make to it. This involves identifying their preferences regarding care and respecting these within the limits of professional practice, existing legislation, resources and the goals of the therapeutic relationship. (NMC, 2004: 5)

There are four further specific obligations connected to the general declaration that nurses are obliged to respect the patient or client (I will now use 'nurses' as shorthand to include the other professional groups covered by the code).

Q. What general declarations and specific obligations exist within the particular code of conduct that you are familiar with?

The extract I have taken from the NMC code partly embodies the internal and external purposes that I have argued codes of conduct possess. It is telling the public that nurses must respect patients and clients. And it is telling nurses themselves that they must engage in such respect. But as I have said, these purposes of intent and standard setting (for the benefit of both public and professionals) cannot be achieved by the code alone. By itself, the code is simply paper and words. To become the powerful tool implied by the purposes I have attached to it, the code needs to be part of what might be called a professional triumvirate (Bowles et al., 2006: 34–35). This triumvirate is formed of these things:

- Statutory professional training;
- Mandatory professional registration;
- The professional code of conduct.

In order to become a registered nurse, to be recognised and practise as such, a person has to undertake a lengthy period of training at an approved institution. This is not optional. I cannot wake up one morning and decide that today I am going to be a nurse. The law requires that I have undergone an approved programme of training before I am able to put myself forward for admission to the list of registered nurses. If I don't pass through these processes yet claim to be a nurse, then I am breaking the law and committing a criminal offence (Department of Health, 1997). Once I am a registered (legal) practitioner, my actions are governed by the standards of conduct determined by the regulatory body for nursing, the NMC. The government (the executive) and the legislature (parliament) delegate to the NMC the task of upholding and developing the professional standards of nursing and midwifery. If a nurse was alleged to have breached the code (say she was accused of clearly failing to respect a patient by telling them lies, or through verbal abuse) and if this allegation was proven, then the nurse would face sanctions and possibly removal from the list of registered practitioners. (Depending on the offence, she might also face criminal or civil prosecution.)

Because of the other two parts of the triumvirate (statutory training and mandatory registration), a code of conduct (in this case, that of nursing) can now meet its purposes. It declares professional intent and the guarantee of standards to the public it serves because it is clear that this is what can be expected from members of the profession. If a particular member fails to meet these standards, sanctions will be applied. It provides guidance and unity for the profession's members because they recognise that they must behave in certain ways in order to avoid the profession coming into disrepute. Moreover, if a particular professional brings disrepute on himself, then he will be faced with removal of his registration and all the consequences that are likely to flow from this (loss of job, livelihood, status, and so on).

Of course, none of this provides a guarantee that professionals (in this case, nurses) will always and in every case act according to the requirements of the code of conduct. In the same way that the simple existence of the general law obviously cannot guarantee that there will be no criminal behaviour in our society, the existence of the code does not mean that nurses will never break it (Revill, 2006a). Given this, the questions that we can most usefully ask at this point are these:

- Does a code of conduct make it more or less likely that a professional will behave ethically?
- Does a code of conduct make it more or less likely that the public to be served by the profession will see it as ethically robust?

Difficulties with Codes of Conduct

We might be able to move towards answering these questions through empirical investigation, through going out and asking people (by means of questionnaires or interviews, say) about their professional or personal experiences. (From Chapter 4, this would form a non-*a priori*, empirical argument.) What I am going to do here, though, is to construct an argument about difficulties with codes of conduct that is broadly, but not strictly, *a priori*. It tries to apply reason to what we know or recognise *generally* about codes and about professional practice in order to reach its conclusions about the difficulties they involve.

Example

Stephen Jacobs is a mental health nurse, working for a mental health care NHS Trust. He has been asked by his managers to monitor restrictions on smoking in a number of wards within the Trust's inpatient facility, following the legal ban on smoking in enclosed public places in England introduced by the government in July 2007 (Department of Health, 2006). On the first of what he intends to be regular monitoring visits, he talks to a number of patients about the ban. They are united in their opposition to it. 'It's forcing us not to smoke when we want to.' 'Why should we have to give up smoking because the government says so?' These are just a couple of the comments that he has picked up. When he points out that the Trust has built special shelters outside the wards where people can go and smoke if they want, the patients become even angrier. 'Forcing us out into the rain! That's what they'd like to do with us permanently if they could get away with it! They just see us as dregs they can do what they like with. They're not interested in us – never have been, never will be.' Staff members join in with the complaints. 'If you were a smoker, how would you feel about the organisation that sent you out into the cold every time you had a break?' Stephen comes away from the visit wondering how he should present his report on the restrictions, which he is due to give to the Trust Health and Safety Committee in a few days' time.

In theory at any rate, Stephen Jacobs has at least two possible courses of action that he can take:

- He can describe the difficulties to the Committee, while emphasising that change is always hard to accept and the restrictions will produce so much benefit that resistance should be listened to politely but essentially ignored. We might call this **the conservative course.**
- He can act as a 'voice' for the angry patients and disillusioned staff, strongly suggesting that the Committee seriously needs to consider and respond to the widespread discontent. This could be called **the radical course.**

In relation to our discussion, the key question we need to ask is this: Can Stephen be helped in making a choice between these two different courses of action by a code of conduct (in this case, the NMC Code)?

The first difficulty: codes as 'inflexible edicts'

There are two aspects of the NMC Code that appear relevant to the situation Stephen faces. Section 3.2 of the Code states: 'You must respect patients' and clients' autonomy – their right to decide whether or not to undergo any health care intervention' (NMC, 2004: 5). While Section 8.1 reads: 'You must work with other members of the team to promote health care environments that are conducive to safe, therapeutic and ethical practice' (NMC, 2004: 11). Stephen believes he is right to interpret the smoking restrictions as a 'health care intervention'. Why else would they have been implemented other than to protect the health of patients and staff? (He recognises that there may well be other reasons, but is prepared at the moment to accept this is the primary motivation of the policy makers.)

These sections of the code suggest two things to Stephen. First, if he takes the conservative course at the Health and Safety Committee, he will not be properly respecting patients' autonomy. They are deeply unhappy with the intervention that has been imposed on them and he will not be allowing proper voice to their frustrations. The patients (and staff) are definitely not saying, 'Well, it's hard, but it always is when you have to cope with change – we'll get used to it.' They simply *don't want* to be restricted in their smoking behaviour. So Section 3.2 of the Code appears to provide justification for the radical course of action. Second, on the other hand, Section 8.1 and its requirement to promote safe and therapeutic health care environments seem to offer support for the conservative course. Which should be taken?

The difficulty here is that, as with the four principles approach I discussed in the previous chapter, there is apparent conflict between separate sections of the Code. To put it in the language of the four principles, are we most interested in respecting autonomy, or in producing benefit? However, this difficulty of conflict between values is even more problematic in the case of codes. The four principles, as I discussed, aim to provide a framework for understanding and allow for judgement and choice when there appears to be competition between them. The NMC Code (along with others, I would argue) does not make that allowance. It simply says: 'You must ... respect the patient or client as an individual ... [and] act to identify and minimise risk to patients and clients' (NMC, 2004: 3).

Clearly, in the example of Stephen Jacobs (along with many others), conflict exists between these two separate requirements yet the Code insists that practitioners must conform to both. In doing so, its character seems to be more that of an 'inflexible edict' than a framework for ethical deliberation.

The second difficulty: codes as expressions of professional belief

Although my phrasing is a bit prejudicial, we may have some sympathy with the idea of codes as 'inflexible edicts', given their purposes of standard setting and declaration of professional intent. After all, the public are probably expecting health care professionals to represent themselves quite definitively. As a member of the public, I want a nurse to say to me, 'If you come to me for help, I will do this.' I would be slightly bemused and possibly alarmed if instead he said, ' If you come to me for help, I will do this. Unless x applies, in which case I would do that. But if y was present I may well do something else.' So it might be possible to argue that codes have to take on a strong and definitive shape if they are to convince health care professions' public audiences. This, however, leads to the second difficulty with codes – that they seem to privilege professional over so-called lay beliefs.

There are many stories behind the ban on smoking in enclosed public spaces that was introduced in England in 2007. (Bans had earlier been imposed in other countries of the British Isles as well as in some other European and overseas countries.) Stephen may or may not have been aware of them. One that seems especially relevant emerged from the House of Commons Health Committee, which in 2005–06 was considering the nature and possible implications of a ban (House of Commons Health Committee (HOCHC), 2006). At one of its sessions, the idea of exemptions to the ban was being considered. The Committee noted that: 'Smoking prevalence among the mentally ill, and especially those who are in some kind of institutional care, is very high' (HOCHC, 2006: 33). This led to the question of whether inpatient mental health facilities should be exempted from the ban. At the time, the pressure group Rethink argued against the ban being imposed on inpatient facilities, saying that it would have a detrimental effect on an already marginalised and vulnerable group of people, who would be forced to engage in highly difficult behaviour change. In opposition, the Royal College of Nursing argued that by *not* imposing the ban and so not providing an impetus for patients to give up smoking, a health inequality (increased prevalence of smoking among people with mental health problems) would be perpetuated and even exacerbated.

> Q. Given the circumstances, do you think it is right to impose the national ban on smoking in public places within psychiatric inpatient facilities? Try to justify the position you take and consider how a code of conduct would help or (hinder) you in moving towards that position.

The HOCHC eventually reached this conclusion on the matter: 'High levels of smoking in psychiatric institutions are not inevitable. ... Psychiatric units should not be granted a simple exemption from the smoke-free provisions of the Health Bill' (HOCHC, 2006: 34). In the Health Act 2006 itself, mental health institutions were granted a little more time to prepare for a ban (arrangements would have to be in place by 1 July 2008 rather than 1 July 2007). The fact remains, though, that Stephen Jacobs' Trust has imposed the restrictions that he has been asked to monitor.

How does this story relate to difficulties with codes of conduct? Stephen is faced with two apparently conflicting elements of the NMC Code, as it seems to apply in this situation: respect patients and their autonomy or act to minimise patient risk. My consideration of the context so far leads strongly to the view that he cannot do both things. But the context actually does more than foster ambivalence. It makes it more likely that Stephen will adopt the conservative course of action (that is, to describe but essentially ignore patient anger about the restrictions). Political and professional judgement, as we have seen in the debates of the House of Commons Committee, have inclined towards the belief that smoking is somehow 'inauthentic' action (Rawson, 1994). It is *not* smoking that is authentic and should therefore be the norm. We might accept this view, but then again we might not. After all, it seems rather disrespectful to suggest that significant numbers of people (including many people with mental health problems) are acting in ways that are not authentic. The NMC Code offers no challenge, or prospect of challenge, to the prevailing professional orthodoxy that certain kinds of health-related actions are inauthentic.

Why is this the case? It is simply because this Code (along with others, I would argue) does not aim at radical critique, or the proposition of radical action. Its aim is to express the 'shared values' of the profession and its regulators. These values are shaped by (and in turn shape) the broader context. Both the broader and the particular professional context appear united in the belief that smoking (at least in public places) is an insupportable and inauthentic action. The Code therefore supports Stephen taking the conservative, rather than the radical, course of action in this example.

At this point, somebody might argue that all I'm doing here is to express *my own* personal belief that codes of conduct do not allow challenges to the orthodoxy. There are two responses to this. First, there is no part of the NMC Code that actually advocates the worth of radical challenge to the *status quo*. Its focus on individual behaviour and responsibility diminishes the possibility of challenge to the context. For example, the nurse 'must adhere to the laws of the country in which [she] is practising' (NMC, 2004: 4). On the other hand, if the practitioner feels they have reason to object to a state of affairs, the Code does not allow their right to do so but instead says, 'You must report to a relevant person or authority, at the earliest possible time, any conscientious objection' (NMC, 2004: 5). The emphasis here is firmly on the *responsibility* of the practitioner to notify an objection to authority rather than their *right* to pursue and develop it. In the example of Stephen Jacobs, the requirement would be for him to tell the Trust of his concerns rather than for him to act on them. In this way, the idea of personal challenge is circumvented.

Second, we might well be happy with the idea of codes emphasising personal professional responsibility rather than the right to action if this is primarily about responsibility to patients or clients. However, we do not need to look very far to realise that professional responsibility is also perceived as existing towards organisations and the profession itself (or other members of the profession) (NMC, 2004). Codes do not necessarily help in any conflict that might occur between responsibility to patients or clients, on the one hand, and to organisations or professions, on the other. This is simply because of the enormous power of these contextual influences. Referral to a code of conduct to resolve questions of practice standards is sometimes useless. Cases such as that of Stephen Bolsin, the young consultant who finally revealed the scandal of the Bristol Heart Babies (Kennedy, 2001), or Graham Pink, the charge nurse who exposed the dangerously inadequate levels of staffing on an elderly care ward (Freedom to Care, 2008) demonstrate this. The fact that such cases of 'whistleblowing' have been legitimised by the Public Interest Disclosure Act 1998 (Royal College of Nursing, 2007) seems to demonstrate an inadequacy in codes of conduct themselves. If codes were powerful enough tools to protect patients through engendering individual professional responsibility, we wouldn't need legislation to protect those professionals whose actions conflict with the interests of others apart from patients. That we do need it is demonstration that codes and their use are shaped by broader and more powerful contexts than simply that of the individual practitioner and her patient or client.

Thinking About...

Consider cases of so-called whistleblowing that you might be familiar with. Reflect on the degree of help (or otherwise) that a code of conduct would have been in exposing irregularity or maintaining professional practice in these cases.

All this leads to a sense that codes of conduct – our representative of 'outside in' ethics – require at one and the same time both *too much* and *too little* of the practitioner. They require too much because they expect the practitioner doggedly to obey inflexible and (as the example shows) perhaps contradictory edicts. They require too little because they do not allow the professional to challenge the broader social and organisational contexts in which he works, and which may well be an important source of ethical difficulty. In terms of our debate about how and why we develop our moral awareness and action, codes seem to prod us in certain directions, then leave us exposed and with little support.

From the 'Outside In' to the 'Inside Out': The Idea of 'Virtuous Lives'

If codes hold problems in terms of their capacity to guide and direct us in 'ethical action', where else should we look? Some philosophers believe that we need to look to ourselves, to the moral capacity that we have within us and that we can learn to develop. This idea draws us towards the field of **virtue ethics**.

Virtue ethics is, in the same way as deontology and consequentialism, a normative ethical theory (that is to say, it argues on the basis of already assumed norms). Some have argued that it has now become a major normative theory of ethics (Stohr, 2006). In fact, the tradition of virtue ethics extends back to Ancient Greece and the philosopher Aristotle (384–322 BC). I have deliberately chosen to separate it from the two other normative theories that we have so far discussed, and delayed its introduction a little. This is partly because in recent times it has often been seen in a different way from deontologist or consequentialist theory. It would perhaps be better to say that it has been neglected or even that attempts have been made to discard it (Macintyre, 1985). Quite why is unclear, although if we think again about the idea of historical times shaping ethical theory (as we did in previous chapters) we might construct an argument based on the post-Enlightenment need for rationality in moral theory, which has caused theories such as deontology and consequentialism to dominate (Cottingham, 2008). Virtue theory, until recently to its detriment, has seen **emotion** and **emotional response** as important features of ethical decision-making and action.

Thinking About...

This is the first time that I have explicitly talked about *emotions* playing a part in how we decide to act in an ethical sense. Consider the extent to which your own ethical decisions are based on your emotions and feelings.

There is a need, however, to be careful about drawing too sharp a distinction between virtue ethics, on the one hand, and deontology and consequentialism on the other. Jennifer Jackson has argued that it is a false dichotomy to suggest that virtue theory is about telling us what it is *good* to do and theories of obligation are about telling us what we *must* do. This is because any consideration of what it is good to do has to involve thought about what our obligations in those circumstances might be (Jackson, 2006: 25–26). It is as strange to think of 'good' independently as it is to think of 'obligations' without reference to anything else. Equally, some try to claim that the distinction between virtue theory and obligations-based theories lies in the fact that the former sees right action in terms of what the actor or agent would do, while the latter would see rightness lying in the definition of the right action. But nor is this agent-centred *versus* action-centred dichotomy right. In Kantian ethics, as I discussed in Chapter 4, much is made of the categorical imperative, obligations driving the rational individual towards performing the right action. However, even in such a strongly obligations-focused theory as Kant's, there is also an important focus on the good will of the agent himself (Stohr, 2006).

Virtue ethics: the doctrine of the mean

If this is the case, then what is distinctive about virtue ethics as opposed to the ethics of obligation? The distinctiveness lies partly, as I have said, in virtue theory embracing emotional responses to action and decisions about action. Connected to this, it also lies in how 'good action' is conceived and how the 'good person' actually comes to perform the 'good action'.

Probably the key tradition within virtue ethics is the Aristotelian. Within this, the idea of the so-called 'golden mean' is central (Russell, 1979). For Aristotle, the 'good action' is one that lies at the mean point between two extremes. Consider the example of 'courage'. A *properly* courageous action is one that falls between the extremes of timidity on the one hand, and foolhardiness on the other. Imagine I am strolling by the river that runs through the town near where I live. Sudden cries and shouts wake me from my daydreaming and I see that a child has fallen into the swiftly flowing water. Now clearly, if I was seized by timidity and did nothing, my inaction would not be regarded as courageous. Equally, if I held out a hand that it would be impossible for the drowning child to reach, while worrying all the time about whether I was going to fall in myself, this too would not constitute courage. On the other extreme, imagine that the child was a split second away from being sucked through a weir and into the low, narrow tunnel that the river passes through at this point. If I jumped in myself to try to save her now, it is almost certain that we would both be drowned. If this actually happened, the local newspaper report on the incident might very well call me a 'hero'. However, in Aristotelian terms, my foolhardiness means that I would not have been properly courageous and my action could not therefore be called 'good'. The child would not have been saved, and I would have been drowned myself. Two valuable lives would have been lost. In this example, the courageous action would have been that which discarded both timidity and foolhardiness and sought the mean between them (say, I jumped into the river to save the child knowing that the risk was great but there was a good chance I could rescue her and a reasonable possibility that I would survive as well).

> Q.• What difficulties do you think there might be with the doctrine of the
> •'golden mean', which is central to many virtue-based accounts of ethics?
> Note your responses to this question.

One fairly clear problem is that of knowing what the 'virtuous mean' might be in any given situation. In the drowning child example above, how could I possibly weigh up what might actually constitute a courageous action in a few dangerous seconds? Even in less pressing situations, we might have great difficulty in conceiving what is a good (virtuous) action in that particular circumstance. The Aristotelian answer to this problem lies in the agent-centred nature of virtue theory (Stohr, 2006). The virtuous agent seeks and undertakes the good (virtuous) action.

However, this answer sounds more than a bit circuitous. The idea that I perform good actions because I'm virtuous doesn't really get us anywhere. Exactly how do I become virtuous? The response to this question from the Aristotelian is that I do so through learning. I learn to become virtuous, to perform the good action, through following example, through observation of others and through reflection on my own experiences. Observation and reflection involves examination of both rational thought (cognition) and, importantly, as I have said, emotion and feeling (affection). In my imaginary drowning child example, as I was making up my mind what to do, I would have been able to draw on rational thought (calculating the dangers present in the situation), emotion (spontaneous sympathy for the terrible plight of the child) and feeling (a desire to act bound with worries about the implications of acting for my own safety and for my family's well-being if anything were to happen to me). For the Aristotelian virtue theorist, the point is that all of this would have taken place naturally because my life up to that point had been preoccupied with learning to live virtuously through following example, and through observation and reflection. As AC Grayling puts it:

> If one cannot be practically wise, says Aristotle, one should imitate those who are. Eventually this has a good chance of helping one learn how to be prudent, for in any case identifying the mean and acting in accordance with it in given situations is a matter of developing habits of practical wisdom, and becoming skilled in ethical judgement. Living the good life is a whole-life project, and accordingly is something in which one can perfect oneself. (Grayling, 2003: 29)

The difficulty with 'virtuous lives'

Returning to the idea I discussed in Chapter 3, the idea that philosophers and their ideas are distinct products of their own social times, we need to be reminded what Aristotle, in his development of the notion of 'virtuous lives', was trying to do. Ancient Greece was ordered according to city-states, in which each citizen (free men, not women or slaves!) was directly part of the governance of the state. It was therefore in the interest of the state to be ruled by virtuous men. In the sense that these men were arbiters and rulers, what was required was the capacity to develop good lives rather than a reliance on prescriptive rules (for who was going to tell the rulers what rules to follow?). Seen in this way, the contrast is clear between the 'inside out' nature of virtue ethics and the 'outside in' character of the other normative ethical theories of obligation that we have examined (and their manifestations in codes of conduct).

But while I have identified major problems with the adequacy of moral guidance provided by codes ('outside in' ethics), there is equally a need to pose a challenge to virtue theory (a representative of 'inside out' ethics). There are two connected elements to the challenge. First, there is the question of the extent to which virtue theory is of practical help in making decisions. Second, there is the issue of how far it is realistic or possible for decisions made by those pursuing 'virtuous lives' to play a part in the problematic and disputed world of health care.

Let's return to the example of Stephen Jacobs and the restrictions on smoking that he is responsible for monitoring in the mental health care Trust for which he works. To what extent will reference to virtue theory in his position of 'piggy in the middle' of patients and staff on one side, and Trust management on the other, help him? The main difficulty seems to be that Stephen's possible actions (the conservative course of neutral reporting to the Trust Committee *versus* the radical one of acting as a 'voice' for disgruntled patients and staff) do not seem to be amenable to analysis and reflection in the light of the doctrine of the 'golden mean'. In the example of the drowning child, it was relatively easy to establish what was the properly courageous action (the mean between timidity and foolhardiness). But what is the mean in the Stephen example? What virtue should we try to attach to it? Are we seeking an action that represents courage in this situation? Honesty? Loyalty? Are we searching for justice? Or are we looking for all of these things? If we are seeking a particular virtue, then there is likely to be conflict between what we are searching for and other things that might equally be regarded as virtuous. For example, the virtue of loyalty (to Stephen's employer, say) might best be served by careful and neutral reporting to the Committee (though it's quite likely that Stephen will consider he also has loyalty to the patients and staff, which might well result in a very different course of action). But if Stephen definitely decided to speak up for the voiceless patients, this might best serve the virtue of justice. Given this, it seems quite clear that trying to serve all the virtues is impossible.

As Stohr (2006: 24) remarks, 'Virtue ethicists are not rushing to defend the idea that virtue ethics can supply a complete decision procedure'. This is not necessarily a bad thing; after all, one of the central criticisms that I have made of codes of conduct and theories of obligation more generally has been that, in driving our decisions in particular directions, they perhaps fail to allow for the nuance and ambiguity contained in many situations. However, the 'decision procedure' offered by virtue ethics seems to be not just incomplete, it gives the impression of being almost hazardously vague. The seeming lack of capacity for supporting practical decision-making leads us to the second component of the difficulty with virtue theory – how far is it realistic or possible for decisions made by those pursuing 'virtuous lives' to play a part in the problematic and disputed world of health care?

Health care requires and demands decision-making, and actions consequent on decisions that have been made. Decisions and action are often taken with limited time for appraisal of the options, and with limited resources available (Cribb, 2005). Decisions are often made at one level, with the expectation that they will be enacted at another (as in the example of Stephen). Dispute, dissent and disagreement are central features of the landscape. (They are key themes of this book *simply because* that is the case.) I argued above that for the Aristotelian virtue theorist, we act virtuously by learning to lead virtuous lives. But in the health care world of limited time and resources, decision-making at different levels, and dispute within and between these different levels, the scope for learning to live the virtuous life through following example, through observation and reflection, is surely limited. Contemporary health care is not ordered in the same way as Aristotle's city-state; the democratic reach (if it exists at all) is much more distant. The two elements of the difficulty with virtue ethics in the health care context – the vagueness in its 'decision procedures' and the complexity of the context in which these vague procedures will have to be applied – combine to cause concern about its applicability. In terms of debate about how and why we develop our professional moral capacity, the focus of virtue theory on the self (in contrast to codes) might be laudable, but in the health care context at least it presents great difficulties.

Thinking About...

Consider how easy (or how hard) it might be to develop a 'virtuous life' in your own health care situation. Think especially about the resources you might need and the extent to which they are (or are not) available to you.

Conclusion: Drawing Together Ethics from the 'Outside In' and the 'Inside Out'

I have argued that understanding the basis of ethical behaviour as emerging from the 'outside in' (through the fierce obligations enshrined in codes of conduct and bestowed on practitioners from on high) poses major problems. Put bluntly, their prescription might allow those involved in practice a licence for 'moral thoughtlessness' through slavish obedience to what are considered to be the rules. Equally, though, as I have just argued, ethics from the 'inside out' poses problems because of its ambitious (and maybe in the contemporary health care context unrealistic) focus on the development of 'virtuous' (good) lives.

To some extent, the division between 'outside in' and 'inside out' ethics is an artificially constructed one, designed to highlight the tensions within and between different conceptions of the basis of ethical behaviour. We would probably agree that as we make decisions and undertake actions, we are guided both by our knowledge of the obligations that we have and by attempts to lead a 'good life' to the best of our ability. Nevertheless, the division is an important one because underlying it are very different values, and very different views on how we should engage in what I will call **moral education**.

By moral education I mean the processes through which we develop our ethical and values-related sensibilities and awareness, and ultimately our capacity to deliberate on situations and make appropriate moral judgements. I do not mean attempts to inculcate particular values or ethical stances (Carr, 2003). If we believe that ethics is imparted from the 'outside in', then our strategies and practices for professional moral education will centre around things like the delivery of knowledge and understanding from accepted canons, most probably by recognised experts. However, if we think that ethics is developed from the 'inside out', our concerns will be much more to do with 'leading out', facilitating and supporting the individual so that they recognise their moral capacity and potential (Peters, 1973).

Again, the practical view is that professional moral education requires both the expert and the facilitator. However, questions remain about the extent to which the expert, on the one hand, and the facilitator, on the other, are involved, as well as about the degree of self-reliance and the resources required for the process of moral education. These are questions that I will return to in the final chapter of this book. For now, with the benefit of the discussions we have so far had about the nature of values- and ethics-related thinking and its grounding, I will move to discuss some of the particular ethical problems facing those involved in health care, especially what I have tended to call 'ordinary' health care.

Chapter Summary

In this chapter, I have:

- Explored the help that codes of conduct (as representatives of 'outside in' ethics) can offer those involved in health care;
- Considered the use of virtue theory and the idea of the virtues ('inside out' ethics) as a way of understanding and engaging in ethical action in health care;
- Developed an account of the difficulties with both 'outside in' and 'inside out' ethics and suggested that we need to engage in further thinking in order to flesh out what we might mean and what we might do in order to engage in our own professional moral education.

Further Reading

Dawson, AJ (1994). Professional codes of practice and ethical conduct. *Journal of Applied Philosophy*, 11, 2, 145–53. This paper provides a valuable discussion of codes of conduct in the context of Dawson's distinction between 'inside out' and 'outside in' ethics.

Grayling, AC (2003). *What is Good? The Search for the Best Way to Live*. London: Wiedenfeld and Nicolson. Grayling, one of the best-known contemporary philosophers in the UK, provides a very readable account of the search for 'the good life'.

7

THE WELFARE OF THE INDIVIDUAL: HEALTH CARE, AUTONOMY AND INFORMED CONSENT

Learning Outcomes

By the end of this chapter, you should be able to:

○ Describe and discuss some of the kinds of health care situations in which ethical questions related to the welfare of the individual are important;
○ Describe and discuss problems connected to autonomy and individual welfare in health care;
○ Describe and discuss the concept of informed consent, as it might be understood in the health care context;
○ Discuss difficulties with the practice of informed consent by those working in health care.

Introduction

Health care is often (perhaps mostly) directed towards restoring, maintaining and improving the health of individuals. I want to argue in this chapter that as they attempt to do so, health care workers face significant ethical challenges. These challenges most frequently centre on questions of individual autonomy. To what extent does (or should) an individual possess autonomy in relation to their health, and health care decisions made about them? Is it right for health care workers to argue in any sense for restrictions in the personal autonomy of their patients or clients? How can patient or client autonomy be protected? This chapter aims to explore some of the ethical dimensions of health care work aimed at individual welfare, and does so mainly through a lens focused on individual relationships between health care workers and their patients or clients. In Chapter 8, the lens is broadened as I consider the connection between individuals involved in health care and the wider health policy context in which they work or are cared for. Here, I will argue, considerations of justice in the health care and policy context become important.

There is a need for caution at this point. The relatively narrow focus of the lens in this chapter and the relatively broader one within the following chapter should not be taken to imply that we are talking about two different things; what might be called 'individual ethics' on the one hand, and 'policy ethics' on the other. Certainly, there are obvious differences involved in exploration of these two kinds of areas. One of the greatest, perhaps, is that the area of 'health policy ethics' has generally been subject to much less exploration than the 'ethics of individual health care' (Cribb, 2005). This is especially so with regard to what we might call public health or health promotion dimensions of health policy (Mittlelmark, 2007).

In planning this book, my original intention was to write two chapters that would clearly demarcate the ethics of individual care from policy ethics, and especially the ethics of public health policy. However, in reading and thinking about the overall content of this part of the book, it became clearer to me that this kind of division would not necessarily be helpful. Many of the issues that I consider in this chapter and the following one – autonomy, conceptions of personhood, rights and justice, persuasion and coercion for health – span both 'individual' and 'policy' ethics. What seems to matter most, and what makes the difference in our perceptions, is the perspective from which we see the issues. We can view them either from the perspective of the practitioner focused on the patient or client, or we can see them from one that looks beyond wards, clinics and individual consultations to the society that provides the context for these. There is a *tendency* for us to see things from the former, narrower perspective. This holds risks. We may think, for example, that the only ethical transaction that is taking place is the one between, say, the physiotherapist and the elderly patient. In doing so, we ignore the social and political backgrounds and context that very importantly frame and feed these transactions. Equally, though, there is risk in *simply* seeing things from the social context and ignoring the 'nitty gritty' of what is going on between the elderly person and the therapist. My final claim, at the end of these two chapters, is that we need to look both *to* our patients and clients as well as *around and beyond* them. I hope the discussions within the chapters will support this claim.

Individual Welfare: Problems of Health Care Practice

The following three examples help to start to tease out some of the ethical difficulties associated with attempts to safeguard, maintain or improve individual welfare as a central part of the health care enterprise. At the core of each, I will argue, are questions of individual autonomy, its preservation and the extent to which it can be respected.

> ### Example
>
> Deborah Humphreys is a health visitor who is involved in running a postnatal support group. One of the group members is first-time mother Michelle Roberts. In the course of several conversations, it becomes clear to Deborah that Michelle is having quite a lot of difficulty in adjusting to motherhood. She has lengthy periods of feeling 'very down' and becomes highly irritable with her partner. 'But I love Daniel [her baby] so much,' she tells Deborah. 'I can't understand it.' In a discussion between Deborah and her line manager, the idea of strongly suggesting to Michelle that she asks her GP to prescribe antidepressant medication comes up. 'Just to get her over the hump,' Deborah's manager says.

A balanced assessment of this situation might include the view that there are good reasons for Deborah to make the suggestion to Michelle and encourage her to seek short-term medication. It may well help her to get over this bad patch. However, there are also doubts about the efficacy of antidepressants in this case of 'mild' depression (although the word 'mild' must be a misnomer to any sufferer) (BBC News, 2008). Deborah has not yet had the discussion with Michelle about taking medication, and of course much depends on her client's reaction when this actually takes place. However, there is at least the possibility of tension as a result of the discussion, with Deborah and Michelle taking different views about the desirability of this approach. Imagine Deborah believes that antidepressants would be helpful and Michelle resists the idea. Regardless of the actual outcome (whether or not Michelle takes the drugs), these different positions represent separate conceptions of what is for the good of the client's welfare and 'in her best interests'. These separate conceptions could potentially lead to alternative views about client autonomy; Deborah believing, say, that strong encouragement and emphasis on the benefit of medication is better than a more neutral discussion in which Michelle's feelings and choices dominate.

> ### Example
>
> James Morris is a 60 year-old man with a history of coronary heart disease (CHD). For most of his adult life, he has been a heavy smoker (at least one packet a day). He is also significantly overweight. He suffers from mobility problems and a left hip replacement has been suggested. However, his local NHS Trust refuses to fund such operations for those who smoke or are overweight (BBC News, 2007).

The example of Mr Morris exposes a rather different dimension to questions of autonomy and individual welfare in health care. Here the difficulty is not one of competing versions of 'welfare' and the effect that this might have on how autonomy is regarded. It is rather that 'welfare' is being restricted, with the consequent disruption of Mr Morris's autonomy. There is no doubt that he will benefit from a hip replacement operation, but because of his current lifestyle he is being denied this benefit. In the view of the NHS Trust, his lifestyle is 'inauthentic' and unless it is changed, he forfeits his right to treatment. The problem can best be seen as one of 'rights'. Does Mr Morris have the right to be both 'unhealthy' (by some accounts) *and* receive state-funded treatment? Does the Trust have the right to deny him treatment? Whatever position is taken, its effect on autonomy (that of Mr Morris or of others) is clear.

Thinking About....

We often talk about rights, and especially about 'human rights' (Wright, 2007). However, such talk is often quite loose and does not recognise the complexity of the concept of 'rights'. We can have *legal rights* (our entitlements under the law at any given time). More problematically, there is the philosophical idea of *moral* (or *natural*) *rights*. Those who assert the existence of moral rights do so from the position that there are just some things which, because we are human, we have a right to (such as health care, perhaps). Others argue that any idea of 'right' is contingent on the particular place and time we happen to be living in. (Our 'right' to health care only exists because we happen to be living in twenty-first-century Britain rather than eighteenth-century Russia.) There is a further distinction to be made between *positive* rights (those that others have a duty to fulfil) and *negative* ones (those that depend only on the non-interference of others (Wright, 2007).

In the light of these distinctions, reflect on what we might mean when we talk about 'rights' in the example of Mr Morris.

Example

Audrey Bell is a 72 year-old woman who has been diagnosed as being in the early stages of senile dementia (Alzheimer's disease). She lives with her husband in the family home of 30 years. Her general practitioner has recently made a social work referral for her. On his first visit the social worker, David Musgrove, is taken aside by Mr Bell. 'I can't cope with her here,' he whispers to David in the hall. 'She'll drive me mad. I know what it's like. I've seen it happen to other people. She has to go into a home.'

In this example yet another dimension in the relationship between autonomy and individual welfare is exposed. Obviously, we would expect David to probe further into the situation and try to establish what it is that Mrs Bell herself actually wants. Imagine, though, that she is adamant she wants to stay in her home. We might possibly be rather concerned with Mr Bell's expression, thinking that somehow he has a duty to look after her until it is impossible for him to do so by himself. However, if we are properly empathetic, we will also be able to understand his position. More than this, we might be inclined to believe that his views about the best place for Mrs Bell are overriding. In this way it is easier to imagine respect for Mrs Bell's autonomy being disrupted (and the disruption being justified through reference to her individual welfare) than it would be in the previous two examples. This is because we can foresee circumstances in which we believe that Mrs Bell would have limited or no control over her own welfare (and what we might call her 'welfare intentions'), so requiring others to step into the situation. In these circumstances, welfare might be prized over autonomy. This is because we might believe (and others may dispute our particular belief) that there are some persons (or classes of persons) whose autonomy we are entitled or obliged to disrupt *just because* they are that kind of person. Samuel Gorovitz (1985: 172) has called these 'cases at the margins of personhood'. Such cases *might* include foetuses, people in persistent vegetative state (PVS) and those with severely diminished mental capacity (Dworkin, 1995).

Personhood and Autonomy

Each of these examples poses very significant problems for health care aimed at individual welfare. We cannot simply say that such activity is ethically unproblematic so long as we take enough care to respect the autonomy of those with whom we are working. Regardless of our professional context or occupation, we are bound to encounter situations where autonomy and its respect are problematic. The examples demonstrate three potential 'threats' to autonomy:

- Competing views about what might produce welfare in a particular situation (Deborah Humphreys and Michelle Roberts);
- Separate ideas on the 'right' to welfare (Mr Morris);
- Different views on the extent to which an individual has the capacity to make feasible choices with regard to her welfare (Mrs Bell).

Each 'threat' is connected to dispute about the extent to which individual autonomy should be 'allowed' in that particular situation. This is connected in turn to the idea that some kinds of persons are able, or should be entitled, to possess more autonomy than others. Underlying all of this is the large philosophical debate about what constitutes a person, and the nature of personhood.

Q. What do you think it is to be a person? Make a note of your responses to this question.

The nature of personhood

The seventeenth-century political philosopher Thomas Hobbes (1588–1679) wrote, ' A person is he, whose words or actions … are considered as his own'

(Sprague, 1978: 24). Contemporary philosophers (Glover, 1977; Gorovitz, 1985) have at one and the same time grounded and extended this notion. Samuel Gorovitz has argued that a person is *at the very least* a sentient being (that is, someone who has awareness of his sensations). But we would surely also want to think of a person as someone who has self-awareness, a capacity for reflection, relationships with others, plans, intentions, aspirations and dreams (Gorovitz, 1985; Sprague, 1978). This in turn leads to the idea that being a person depends on our capacity to apply what philosophers talk of as 'personal predicates' to ourselves and to others. These are words like doing, trying, intending, thinking, feeling, and so on (Sprague, 1978). I can say of myself that I am doing (or thinking) or whatever and I can say the same of other people. On this account, the ascription of personhood to another (through our application of personal predicates to her) is what makes her a person (Sprague, 1978: 72).

This position leads to what Dworkin (1995: 23) calls the use of 'the person' in 'the practical sense'. A person is someone who has a right to be treated as a person because she is someone like you or me, who are undeniably persons (because we think and feel and have plans and intentions).

One central difficulty with this idea, in terms of our discussions on health care as it relates to the welfare of individuals, is that it does not really get us very much further in dealing with our chosen examples. If we believe that a person is somebody who can be described in terms of personal predicates and can offer such a description of others, two key questions are raised:

- Do we have to do or be all of these things (or more) in order to be considered a person?
- Is there one thing on this list of things making up a person that is the one *essential* feature of personhood?

Let's think carefully about the first question. It will be possible to apply only a limited number of the personal predicates we have listed to a babe in arms, say. She will not have intentions or plans. Thinking and feeling in this kind of case will have much more limited senses than is likely to be so with a fully-grown adult. We might reasonably talk of a baby having the potential for full possession of the range of personal predicates, but this is rather different from thinking that she has these now.

This leads us to the idea that we acquire the things that make us persons over a period of time (Glover, 1977). A baby will grow into a toddler, then a child, an adolescent and finally an adult. In this life course, the things that constitute personhood will develop. For example, while a baby cannot be said to have intentions or plans, a child of eight or nine very often does ('I want to play for Manchester United'). As time carries on, planning becomes more reflective and sophisticated ('I'm not actually that good at football, but I'm very good at playing the violin, so perhaps I should train to be a classical musician'). It follows that if we acquire features of personhood at different periods of time, we can also lose them, and lose them at different times.

But does this mean that there are periods where we are more or less of a person? We would not want to talk, presumably, of a tiny baby not being a person, nor would we want to speak of a very elderly adult in this kind of way. A big part of the reason for this is because, in answer to the second question, it is difficult (I would argue that it is impossible) to identify one single *essential* feature of personhood. Not only is it difficult, it is also dangerous. If we look at recent history, the Nazis believed that the one essential feature of being *a person* was to be racially Aryan, which led to untold and indescribable human misery, including attempts to wipe out an entire other race (Burleigh, 2001).

The relationship between personhood and autonomy

So we fall back to the conclusion that personhood entails possessing some of the features of being a person, along with being able to ascribe it in some way to others. I suggested before that this does not move us very far forward in dealing with our chosen examples. However, it does now enable us to understand them better. If we believe in the 'range of features but no single essential feature' argument for the nature of personhood, it helps us to recognise the reason for the heavy dispute that is likely to be involved in different responses to the examples. Let's say that somebody believed the capacity for rational thought was the essential feature of personhood. We could very easily argue with them that this excludes many (such as young babies) about whom we would be alarmed at their being deprived of the status of persons. Our opponent would then be obliged to amend their position to one in which the capacity for rational thought became an important (but not the essential feature) of personhood. So we could argue (as philosophers frequently do) about this or any other proposed feature of being a person.

Q: How does this understanding affect our view of the examples of Michelle Roberts, Mr Morris and Mrs Bell?

It seems to me that this view underlines the need to be very circumspect about our decisions and actions in each of these cases. I argued before that each of the examples demonstrates a particular 'threat' to the autonomy of the individual concerned (differing views on authentic action, the 'right' to welfare and the capacity for choice-making). The threat is exercised because we think we might be entitled to believe that in the case concerned we can in some way interfere with what the individual wants to do, or what they want to happen. Let's continue for a while to argue with our imagined opponent, the person who believes strongly in the capacity for rational thought as an important feature of personhood. (As I have claimed, she cannot argue that it is the one essential feature of being a person.) Her argument for interference, for autonomy disruption, might well be centred on the idea that in each of these cases the capacity for rational thought, an important feature of being a person, is not present or is not being used. Therefore we have the right to intervene for at least two reasons:

- To save the person concerned from being harmed by their lack of this particular feature of personhood (the **saving from harm principle**);
- To ensure that others are not harmed by the lack of this particular feature on the part of the person concerned (the **saving others from harm principle**).

But do we in fact have a right to intervene (and so disrupt autonomy) in either or both of these respects?

Paternalism, disrupting autonomy and saving from harm

As I discussed in Chapter 5, the corollary of saving from harm is the production of benefit (at least in some regard). Characteristically, efforts to save from harm and so produce benefit are viewed as depending on a belief that others (those doing the saving) have greater insight than we do (the unwitting or conscious indulgers in harm) into what is in our own best interests. Frequently, this belief forms the basis of a divide between patients or clients, on the one hand, and health care workers (or government and policy makers) on the other. The former groups (patients or clients) are seen for one reason or another as lacking understanding of what they should do, while the latter (health care workers and policy makers) possess such understanding and need to act to protect the interests of those whom they are supposed to be serving.

The idea of having greater insight or knowing better than somebody else what is in his own interests is not unusual. It is something that happens all the time in the relationship between parents and their children. Parents frequently assume that they know what is best and act accordingly. This often involves restrictions on apparent freedoms and autonomy ('No, you're not going out now because it's nearly dark and I'm worried about you getting back home safely'). We readily accept such paternalistic restrictions in society, generally licensing parents to act in this kind of way and becoming angry when erstwhile mothers and fathers neglect or do not accept this licence. The question is whether such paternalism can be justified in relationships *between adults* (here between patients or clients on the one hand, and health care workers on the other) (Wikler, 1978).

Q. Paternalism is the overriding of a person's autonomy for the sake of what we assume to be her own interests, to save her from harm and in some way to produce benefit (Glover, 1977: 75). We accept (even encourage) paternalism in relationships between parents (or other carers) and children. Why might paternalistic relationships between health care workers and their patients or clients be much more problematic?

There are at least two reasons why in general we might be concerned about paternalism in health care. First, we tend to work in the social context with the assumption that other people usually know better than ourselves what is right for them, and they don't require us to force them into particular courses of action (Wikler, 1978). This is partly what underscores the essential importance of the principle of respect for autonomy in health care, as I discussed in Chapter 5. Second, health care as an enterprise has great potential to disrupt autonomy, either knowingly or unwittingly. Health care workers do things and do them in ways that we wouldn't ordinarily allow anybody else to do. Who else, for example, would I allow to burrow deep into my mouth other than my dentist? Who but my GP would I willingly allow to question me about my emotional state? (Gorovitz, 1985).

It is possible to understand paternalism as having different forms (Wikler, 1978, 1987). There is what could be called **weak paternalism**. Here, a health care worker might offer moderate or even fairly strong encouragement or advice to a patient to adopt or agree to a particular course of action. In the examples we have been discussing, we might imagine Deborah Humphreys acting in this kind of paternalistic way with Michelle Roberts. Such action could well have a fair degree of ethical acceptability to us. After all, we might argue that Michelle, because of her circumstances, has temporarily lost some of her capacity for competent self-direction and Deborah's intervention will be of help in eventually restoring this. In that way, weak paternalism can be seen as a support for the development and maintenance of personhood and saving Michelle from harm. However, there is also what we might call **strong paternalism**. This can be taken to involve coercion (rather than simply encouragement) and might even include force (of physical, emotional, legal or other kinds). We could argue that strong paternalism is being exercised in the example of Mr Morris. He is being deprived of access to health care (the hip replacement operation) because of his current health status and behaviour. In this case, the ethical acceptability of the NHS Trust's action might appear very dubious to us. This is partly because we understand it as force and deprivation and, as such, its contribution to developing and maintaining Mr Morris's personhood is highly suspect, not to mention its potential for putting him at risk from harm. However, there is a need to note that a version of the saving others from harm principle might be used here to justify the application of strong paternalism. If Mr Morris is allowed his operation, he may well be depriving others of access to treatment, and these others may be more deserving because they do not have his long history of risky behaviour.

> ### Thinking About...
>
> Consider whether either of the forms of paternalism we have discussed might be appropriate to exercise in the three examples of Michelle Roberts, Mr Morris and Mrs Bell.

Informed Consent: How Far Can We Go?

I hope that discussions so far will have yielded a strong sense that the disruption of autonomy in the health care context is highly problematic. It is problematic because of the context itself as well as because of the variety of ways in which we can interpret 'harm' (given that its avoidance, along with the corollary of benefit production, is the justification usually given for interfering). Moreover, weight rests against any question of disrupting autonomy by virtue of the notion of personhood that we have developed, and our natural inclination to leave people to their own devices as much as possible.

Yet at the same time we frequently require health care to operate on the very boundaries of what might be seen as autonomy disruption, and sometimes we even appear to allow it actually to cross these boundaries (Gorovitz, 1985). This problem of those involved in health care potentially playing fast and loose with individual autonomy is very often met by emphasising the importance to practitioners of **informed consent**.

Q.• What do you understand by the idea of informed consent in the health
•care context?

The doctrine of informed consent is widely held and promulgated by health care workers and by the bodies representing them. The Nursing and Midwifery Council Code of Conduct, for example, contains the following statement: 'You must ... obtain [informed] consent before you give any treatment or care' (Nursing and Midwifery Council, 2004: 3).

The doctrine of informed consent is at once both reassuring and troubling. It is reassuring through its apparent simplicity and the potential it has to overcome all kinds of ethical problems related to health care's efforts to maintain and extend individual welfare:

> Physicians [and other health care workers] do the sorts of things to their patients [or clients] that people in general cannot justifiably do to one another. If the patient understands what the physician [or other health care worker] proposes to do and, thus informed, consents to its being done, then the medical [or other kind of health care] intervention is not imposed on the patient in violation of the patient's autonomy; rather, that medical intervention is properly viewed as a service provided to the patient at the patient's request. (Gorovitz, 1985: 38)

However, the doctrine is also troubling because, as Gorovitz discusses, we know that despite this clear-sighted theoretical expression, the practical acting out of informed consent is much more problematic (Cribb, 2005).

Thinking About...

Think of an instance from your own occupational or personal experience where you have been involved in either gaining or giving 'informed consent'. Consider and reflect on what was involved in the process as well as the extent to which it matched Gorovitz's theoretical description above.

The trouble with informed consent

In thinking about your own particular experience of informed consent, you might have come to the conclusion that there is so much that could (and perhaps often does) go wrong with the process. Did I give (or was I in full possession of) all the relevant facts? Did I understand (or did I convey the understanding) that the situation might be subject to change? Did I have (or did I allow) time to think before adding (or encouraging) signature of the consent form? The possibility of error is perhaps not so surprising when the complexity of the process is considered. Informed consent actually involves *two* parallel and connected processes:

- **Informing** (telling the patient or client what will happen, or what is likely to happen);
- **Consenting** (eliciting the agreement of the client or patient to this happening) (Gorovitz, 1985).

I need to emphasise my use of the word 'processes', because both informing and consenting should be understood as continuous, throughout the period of a treatment, intervention or period of care. Perhaps we have a tendency to believe that 'informed consent' is a single event – the act of the patient signing a form following a brief explanation by the health care worker, say, or one instance of verbal agreement. But this cannot be so, simply because of the dynamic nature of health care, and of patients' responses to the enterprise. Let's return for a moment to the example of Michelle Roberts, whose health visitor Deborah Humphries is thinking about whether to encourage her to take antidepressant medication to help with the difficult postnatal feelings that she is experiencing. Imagine that Deborah decides to offer this encouragement. She sits down with Michelle and explains to the best of her ability both the benefits and the drawbacks in taking the medication. Deborah is a conscientious health care professional, so her explanation is as balanced and realistic as it would be reasonable to hope for. Despite this, it is possible that Michelle won't completely understand what is being said to her. There are at least two potential reasons for this. First, the subject of antidepressant therapy is enormously complex (Bower et al., 2006). What works and doesn't work relates not only to medication use but also to how this fits in with other aspects of treatment and care. It is almost certainly likely to be difficult for Michelle to understand this (as well as, perhaps, for Deborah to convey it). This is not simply a question of ignorance or inability, because the second reason for misunderstanding is that Michelle's capacity to take on board explanation may well be limited by the fact that she is very likely to be anxious about her situation, and anxiety invariably affects health care communication (Gorovitz, 1985).

Remember now my earlier claim that the components of informed consent (informing and consenting) are continuous processes. Imagine that on the basis of Deborah's explanation, among other things, Michelle decides to take the antidepressants. Doing this will, in itself, change her situation one way or another, *but things will change anyway*. Say that managing the baby becomes easier because her partner takes on a more active role, or it gets more difficult because the child contracts some kind of illness. Any of this, and much more, will affect Michelle's capacity to cope. At this stage, consent should be renegotiated.

Such negotiation and renegotiation needs to take place right through the period of Michelle's treatment.

Informed consent: from limits to possibilities

Yet belief and experience tell us that such a process of continuous negotiation seldom takes place in health care. More often than not 'consent' boils down to signing a piece of paper after a quick (and possibly vague) explanation, or a casual exchange of words. To say this is not in any way to condemn health care workers. Uniformly, they are busy people and the kind of careful process that I have described is highly demanding and costly. It is costly in terms of both the time that it takes and of the skills and sensitivities that it requires from practitioners (Gorovitz, 1985). The apparent mismatch between the theoretical, ideal notion of informed consent that I have been building up and the hard-pressed reality of those working in health care seems significant. Surely, we must simply do what we can to try to enact a realistic version of informed consent? This in itself should show due regard for problems of autonomy and individual welfare in the health care context; to ask for anything more would be unreasonable.

It is easy to understand this practical request. It is also possible to agree with it, while at the same time not making less of the idea that the doctrine of informed consent is an important protection for both practitioners and their patients or clients against the risk of autonomy disruption. As Gorovitz (1985) notes, patient or client understanding of a particular procedure, treatment or intervention does not need to be perfect. (It's unlikely that it could be, given the complexity of most health care and its dependence on any number of variables.) However, the fact that knowledge and understanding is imperfect does not necessarily mean that it will be inadequate (Gorovitz, 1985: 42). Surely, what is important is that the knowledge provided and the understanding gained is suitable in the context concerned and that it meets the needs of the patient or client. Coupled with this is the idea that one crucial skill health care workers need to have is that of being able to assess the level of understanding that their patient has of the situation she is in and whether this is enough to help in decision-making that can be properly regarded as autonomous. This leads to the idea that it might be possible to develop a practical 'check list' for informed consent, which acknowledges the busy nature and complexity of the health care context, yet which also encourages a sensitivity to the individual in that context, and the potential vulnerability of her autonomy.

Thinking About...

From discussion so far, a 'check list' for informed consent might include the following:

- What level of understanding (of his position and of the proposed intervention) does the patient have at present?
- Is this level of understanding adequate to help the patient make reasonable decisions for himself?

- If not, what extra knowledge, information or support needs to be provided?
- Can this be provided from existing resources? If these can't be identified, what additional resources are required?

Reflect on this embryonic list and consider what, if anything, you would want to have added to it.

Conclusion: From Individual Welfare to the 'Public Health'

I began this chapter with three examples, each of which exposed threats to the disruption of individual autonomy; cases where what I have talked of as health care's general aim to maintain, restore or improve individual welfare might conflict with particular interests in certain situations. Threats emerged from competing views on what might produce welfare (Michelle Roberts), on the 'right' to welfare (Mr Morris) and on the capacity for welfare-related choices (Mrs Bell). At the heart of each of these examples are questions of personhood. If we believe, as I have argued, that there are multiple features, but not one *essential* feature of being a person, and if we also believe that an important part of being a person is acting autonomously and having our autonomous choices respected, then we must be very careful about our grounds for autonomy disruption. It cannot be done in the belief that a patient might make the 'wrong' choice (Michelle Roberts) or that they have made 'poor' choices in the past (Mr Morris). Nor can it be done on the grounds that the person concerned is incapable of choice (Mrs Bell).

In each of these examples (and in many others within health care, I would want to claim), a clear account of the highly difficult doctrine of informed consent will make a difference in helping us decide how to react and what to do. In the case of Michelle Roberts, if we can help her to develop a good enough understanding of the implications of agreeing (or not) to antidepressant medication, her choice is likely to be as autonomous as possible. For Mrs Bell, focusing on her levels of understanding, along with those of her husband (of her current position, of the likely progress of her condition, and so on) will help to establish what is reasonable in terms of autonomy of choice at the present time. And in each case the focus on *client* understanding will guard against the dominant interpretation of 'reasonable' being that of the health care worker.

Perhaps the most difficult example to account for in the light of this discussion is that of Mr Morris. Here, his autonomy has already been restricted, and this restriction has been decided at a distant, organisational level (in contrast to the other two cases). Even so, the discussion in this chapter should have led us to believe that there is nothing related to Mr Morris's personhood (the choices he has made and the actions he has performed) that *in itself* justifies present restrictions on his autonomy. He has not denied an essential feature of personhood (because its features are multiple and contested). Thus we cannot treat him as less of a person and argue on this ground for restrictions to his autonomy. We might possibly be able to argue for restrictions on the basis of accounts of justice in health care, and these could dovetail with what we may regard as the broad institutional or organisational climate in which conceptions of 'consent', 'autonomy' and 'personhood' are developed. This is somewhat in contrast to the individual level that has provided the main focus for the lens through which the questions raised in this chapter have been viewed. There is now a need to turn attention to this broader level, the level of community and society. We need to think about how some of the issues so far raised could play themselves out in a wider context.

Chapter Summary

In this chapter, I have:

- Described and discussed some ethical difficulties associated with health care oriented towards the welfare of the individual;
- Related these to philosophical accounts of the key concepts of personhood and autonomy;
- Offered a critique of the doctrine of informed consent (often seen as health care's catch-all saviour from accusations of autonomy disruption);
- Attempted to suggest how the doctrine might be strengthened in practice.

Further Reading

Campbell, AV (1990). Education or indoctrination: the issue of autonomy in health education. In Doxiadis, S (ed.), *Ethics in Health Education*. Chichester: Wiley. Although its focus is mainly on autonomy in the field of health education, Campbell's discussion is generally useful in helping to form ideas about personhood and autonomy.

Gorovitz, S (1985). *Doctors' Dilemmas: Moral Conflicts and Medical Care*. New York: Oxford University Press. This book contains a very useful discussion of the idea and practice of the doctrine of informed consent.

8

THE WELFARE OF THE PUBLIC: JUSTICE, RESOURCES AND HEALTH POLICY

Learning Outcomes

By the end of this chapter, you should be able to:

o Identify, describe and discuss key ethical difficulties associated with attempts (through policy and other means) to maintain and improve public welfare;
o Describe and discuss conceptions of justice and how they might be employed and understood in the health care and policy context;
o Critically assess strategies (and problems with strategies) for the allocation of health care resources.

Introduction

Mr Morris, the 60 year-old man being denied surgery because of his lifestyle, represents at least two classic questions facing those with responsibility for developing health policy and in doing so maintaining and improving overall public welfare. First, can it ever be reasonable to 'force' people towards health? Second, is it ever possible to decide that some people have greater right to health care resources than others? A cluster of further questions flow from these initial ones. What do we understand by 'force'? Are some kinds of force acceptable and others not? Whose version of health should guide our actions? What do we mean by 'rights' and especially rights in health care? Can there even *be* a right to health care? This chapter aims to explore these questions.

We have come across some of them already (for example, in Chapter 7 we briefly explored the idea of 'rights'). However, it is important to emphasise that discussion in this chapter will take a different turn. This is simply because I am trying to look at the problems they raise through a different lens with a wider focus. I am trying to examine issues from a macro – rather than the micro – level that has often been the focus of my argument and discussion so far. If we think of the example of Mr Morris, say, at the macro-level (what we might call the level of public welfare), we will start to expose quite different tensions and difficulties than if we look at it from the perspective of the individual.

> Q.•Why do you think we might see the example of Mr Morris and denial of
> •treatment in a different way if we are viewing it from a *macro* – rather
> than a *micro* – level? Note your response to this question.

One of the most straightforward answers to the question is that by moving to the broader level, we are exposing ourselves to a much wider set of claims of interest in the matter (Cribb and Duncan, 2002). Previously, our key concern was in establishing and considering the claims of Mr Morris himself with regard to his individual autonomy and welfare. Now we need to pay attention to the claims of others in trying to establish whether denial or access to treatment in his case will benefit what I am calling the public welfare. Relevant others in this particular case might include those whose treatment would be delayed or cancelled because of the priority given to Mr Morris, the health care workers and managers who daily have to handle and make judgements about the use of health care resources, as well as the policy makers and politicians who decide on resource allocation and priority-setting. All of these people will perhaps (in some cases maybe definitely) have different views about the legitimacy of Mr Morris's claims. I suggested in the previous chapter that there is no doubt he will benefit from treatment, and so presumably wants it, but does he have a right or entitlement to it?

This leads us back to the two questions with which I began this chapter. Imagine that a manager in the NHS Trust responsible for providing access to treatment for Mr Morris is reviewing his case. She may make (or more likely may be implementing) a policy judgement that unless he loses weight and stops smoking, he will not be eligible for surgery. But is this coercion towards a particular version of 'health' ethically acceptable? Again, imagine a gathering in some grand ministerial office of the Secretary of State for Health, her ministers and policy advisers. They are attempting to agree on the implementation by the Department of Health (DOH) of policy across England with regard to access to IVF (in vitro fertilisation) treatment for couples unable to conceive. This is currently a matter for individual Primary Care Trusts (PCTs) to decide, with consequent wide variations in access to treatment dependent on geographical location (Ryan, 2006). One of the ideas floated in the meeting is that in order to meet the cost of expanded and uniform provision of IVF, those like Mr Morris, who continue to engage in 'risky' health behaviour, should equally uniformly be denied their treatment. The ethical question, then, is whether childless couples have greater right to health care resources than 'health risk takers'. Of course the two questions (of coercion and of right) are strongly connected. Their connection is partly through the idea of justice. We may believe that justice will be served if Mr Morris and others like him are coerced into a particular version of healthy behaviour in order that scarce health care resources are not wasted. We may consider that justice will be met by prioritising the right to health care of non-risk-taking childless couples over obese smokers. But both of these beliefs about what policy should be agreed or enacted to promote and improve overall public welfare are based on values. As always, if our thinking is to be rigorous, we need to assess the legitimacy of these values.

Public Welfare, Policy and Values

The political scientist David Easton has famously described political policy as 'the authoritative allocation of values' (Easton, 1953: 123). Given that our concern is with health care and health policy as a means to maintaining and improving public welfare, we can assume that health-related policy represents values allocation with regard to health (and thus public welfare) maintenance and improvement. However, it is important to make the following points:

- Much (if not all) public policy has an effect on health (either negative or positive) and therefore on public welfare (Cribb and Duncan, 2002). Say, for example, that as part of its transport policy the government decides to tax all workplace car parking spaces, spend the revenue raised on improving public transport and thus reduce traffic congestion, pollution and accidents. We can certainly say that this policy will affect public welfare but it is not 'health policy'. So we need to distinguish between health and other kinds of policy that will affect welfare. As a matter of fact this probably means all state-sponsored policy, as no government would be so brave as to claim that what it was doing did not affect (positively, it would doubtless argue) public welfare;
- Policy as the 'authoritative allocation of values' takes place across the range of areas that society (most often through government) has an interest in regulating, defending and promoting (for example, economic development, foreign affairs, internal security, and so on). We need to recognise therefore that values allocation is likely to involve competition in at least two different ways. First, between those holding separate conceptions of the value of health (for example, 'medical model' versus 'social model' of health), each believing that what they want to do will produce the best results according to their preferred model. Second, between those holding separate views on what, from the range of potential policy areas, might actually produce the most 'health' (for example, more health care facilities versus maximum possible economic performance).

> ## Thinking About...
>
> Consider and reflect on how Easton's view of political policy as 'the authoritative allocation of values' might help us to understand what is happening in the case of Mr Morris and the denial of treatment.

Justice, Rights and Needs in Health Care

One way of interpreting Mr Morris's case now is to suggest that the policy makers view the best way of maintaining public welfare as being through the denial of his individual treatment. This sounds paradoxical, but we can guess at their logic:

- If Mr Morris is allowed treatment in his present state, it will produce only limited benefit for him as an individual, and then only for a short period of time;
- The resources not spent on Mr Morris could be allocated elsewhere, in which case the benefit will be substantial and long-lasting;
- Therefore, as things stand, Mr Morris should be denied treatment.

Let's leave aside empirical questions such as the extent to which it is possible to be precise in the belief that the resources not used to help Mr Morris will *actually* be used to the kind of effect we imagine elsewhere (Ham, 2004). The ethical question is one of fairness and justice. Is it just to deny Mr Morris treatment for the sake of (unknown) others?

Conceptions of justice in health care

In Chapter 5, I considered the principle of concern for justice as part of a review of the so-called 'famous four' principles of health care ethics. I described three elements within a concern for justice in the health care context. These are **distributive justice** (concern for fair distribution of scarce health care resources), **natural justice** (concern that our natural moral entitlements are met) and **legal justice** (concern that obligations and entitlements meet the requirements of the governing law).

> Q. Which element (or elements) of the principle of concern for justice might be involved in the example of Mr Morris and denial of treatment?

It does not seem easy to associate the example with a concern for meeting legal justice. While legal frameworks – Acts of Parliament, amendments to Acts and regulations – govern the NHS, the general legal duty on the part of government to provide health care is remarkably vague. Section 3(1) of the NHS Act 1977 (Department of Health and Social Services, 1977) requires the Secretary of State to provide health services to the extent he considers necessary to 'meet all reasonable requirements'. Despite a plethora of 'rights' related to treatment and care set down by successive governments in so-called Patients' Charters and the like, these cannot be seen as legal entitlements. Rather, they are policies supposedly designed to support health service development and embody attempts by policy makers to recognise rising public expectations of the Health Service (Ham, 2004: 85). Even the Human Rights Act 1998, which enshrined the European Convention on Human Rights into UK domestic law for the first time and which includes articles such as the Right to Life, does not provide legal guarantees that particular demands for treatment or care will be met. An example of this is the case of Dianne Pretty, who was dying from motor neurone disease and seeking the right to be assisted towards death. Both the House of Lords and then the European Court of Human Rights judged that the fact that assisted suicide was a crime did not breach Mrs Pretty's human rights (*Guardian*, 2002). Given all this, it doesn't seem possible definitively to associate the claims of Mr Morris (or the rejection of those claims by the NHS Trust) with conceptions of legal justice. The legal framework is so general and, in consequence, the courts, as I mentioned earlier, tend to be reluctant to overturn the judgements of health care providers (Duncan, 2008).

Yet bearing strongly in mind Jennifer Jackson's claim that considerations of justice are 'indispensable' in discussions related to health care ethics (Jackson, 2006: 41), can we relate the claims and counter-claims in Mr Morris's case to the other conceptions of justice that I have mentioned – distributive and natural rights-based justice?

Natural rights and health care

Thinking About...

Review the description of 'rights' on page 65 before reading the following section.

What is the connection between justice and rights? What exactly do we mean when we talk of 'natural rights'? Let me take the first question. When we talk about somebody having a right to something, what we mean is that the person is entitled to the thing (whatever it is) and the thing is due to her (Buchanan, 1984). I make an agreement with my daughter that I will give her pocket money every week. Therefore she is entitled to receive this weekly pocket money; it is her due and her **right**. If I deny her the pocket money, **justice** will be damaged. But say that apart from not giving my daughter pocket money, I also want a 40-inch flat-screen television. Quite clearly I do not have a right and an entitlement to such a thing (unless I have paid the money to the electrical store to supply me with one, which I haven't) and so it is not due to me. Justice is therefore not being breached by life's failure to supply me with the flat-screen TV.

In the pocket money example above, although we may talk most naturally about my daughter's right to the cash being embodied in some kind of contractual right, it might also be possible to argue it is actually a **natural right** that is being breached. There are two possible arguments, based on the 'negative' and 'positive' rights distinction I drew in the previous chapter:

- My daughter has the natural right to freedom from a tyrannical parent who deprives her of pocket money (a **negative right**);
- My daughter has the natural right to freedom of access to the particular resource of weekly pocket money (a **positive right**).

My emphasis on freedom (obviously included in which we can count such things as autonomy and self-rule) in these arguments is quite deliberate. This is because frequently in philosophy a close connection is made between rights and **liberty** (freedom) (Plant, 2002). As is the case with rights, a philosophical distinction has been drawn between **negative liberty** on the one hand (**freedom from**), and **positive liberty** on the other (**freedom to**) (Berlin, 2002).

> Q: What freedoms do you think a patient (or potential patient) entering the health care system is entitled to? Make one list of entitled negative freedoms (freedoms *from*) and another of entitled positive freedoms (freedom *to*).

For myself, imagining my entry as a patient into the health care system (say, I have a persistent cough that won't go away), it is fairly easy to construct a list of negative freedoms that I am entitled to possess. I should be free from intimidation or coercion, free from immediate financial charges (given that I am entering the NHS, which is funded from general taxation and without cost at the point of delivery), free from professionals making assumptions about my physical state or lifestyle, and so on. All such negative freedoms are fundamentally important to our experience as patients and we probably think about them only rarely, if ever (unless of course they happen to be breached).

It is much harder to construct a list of positive freedoms as I enter the NHS with my worrying symptoms. Do I have freedom to choose the hospital I attend for specialist investigations? The consultant I am referred to? The actual diagnostic tests that I undergo? The nurses who look after me? I may have preferences with regard to all of these things but, despite political rhetoric, much 'choice' (freedom) in health care is illusory, partly because of the constantly unpredictable demands placed on the system (I may turn up for an appointment with my preferred consultant only to find that she has been whisked away to perform emergency surgery on somebody else) (Bradshaw and Bradshaw, 2004). We usually find ourselves accepting such limitations on our potential positive freedom (in current political terms, our 'choice') in health care (unless things are going badly awry) for very good reason, as I will argue when we consider distributive justice in health care. However, this assessment of the negative and positive freedoms we feel that we may or may not have as health care patients leads to an important question: Exactly what kinds of natural or moral rights do we have with regard to health care, especially rights related to positive liberties, which I have asserted are particularly hard to identify? (Plant, 1989).

This is a critical question for Mr Morris. As I have argued, it is very unlikely that a case could be made for him having a legal entitlement to the treatment he is being denied. But does he have a moral or natural right to it? With a little recasting of the rather trivial pocket money argument that I introduced before, we can consider two possible arguments for the natural rights of Mr Morris to treatment:

- He has the natural right to freedom from the burden of continuing disease, discomfort and pain that not being treated would lead to (the negative right);
- He has the natural right to freedom of access to the particular treatment he is seeking (the positive right).

It is important to note that I can agree with the first (negative) right without necessarily agreeing to the second (positive) one. Moreover, I want to argue that it is rather easier to construct and agree to an argument in support of the first right than it is to an argument in support of the second. From our discussions in Chapter 7, we developed an account of personhood in which autonomy (the capacity for deliberated self-rule) was central. If we restrict Mr Morris's autonomy by not treating him, then we are placing limits on his natural negative right to freedom from autonomy disruption. However, this does *not* mean we agree that he should receive the treatment concerned. All it means is that we should consider what we might need to do in order to remove the restrictions currently placed upon him.

This is because any positive rights to liberty in health care treatment and care that we might have must, in the same way as our negative rights, be circumscribed by beliefs about what it is to be a person. To be a person, we believe, is in part to be free. An important element of freedom is the capacity for choice and agency, and the well-being and autonomy that are its foundations (Plant, 2002). Our right to positive freedoms with regard to health care, then, must be related to the extent to which they help us retain and maintain this capacity. This is not the same as saying that we have a positive right to limitless health care choices. Such a claim would be foolhardy. It would be foolhardy partly because in trying to make it we would actually be ignoring the natural rights of many others.

Given this, does Mr Morris have the right to hip replacement surgery, presently denied to him because of Trust policy? In support of this particular right, we can say that allowing the surgery will help retain his positive capacity for choice and agency. The freedom allowed therefore corresponds with a reasonable view of personhood. However, it could also be argued that by smoking and being overweight (and this state of affairs quite possibly continuing), the surgery will *not* actually help Mr Morris's capacity. (The treatment will be relatively ineffective, he will quickly become immobile again, and so on.)

In this case, there is no reason to approve the surgery because it will make no difference to his freedom and personhood. Approving it will also (at least potentially) affect the natural rights of others who might as a result be denied treatment that *will* in fact benefit their capacity for choice and agency (childless couples seeking IVF treatment, for example).

The problem is this. Within the rubric that we logically cannot have limitless choices and resources in health care (or any other aspect of life), we are partly circumscribed by the choices that we do in fact make. They help to define us as persons. They may also alter our claims on, and entitlements to, resources. Equally, there are constraints we face that affect the claims we might place on health care resources, or our capacity to make such claims. These would include such things as, for example, constraints imposed as a result of my ethnicity, or gender, or social class (Dougherty, 1993). The question now is one of determining how we can account for both free choice and constraint and come to a reasonable view about entitlement to health care resources, not only for individuals but also for communities and populations, and ultimately the public welfare. Such determining should, we can reasonably argue, underpin policy decisions on resource allocation. We are being led towards thinking about need and distributive justice.

Health care need and distributive justice

The decision we seem to be moving towards with regard to Mr Morris's natural right to the treatment that he is seeking may make us rather uncomfortable. Although we might agree in a rational sense with the policy argument supporting it, emotionally we may be appalled at the thought of somebody continuing to suffer through their being denied treatment.

Q.How would you deal, both as a health care worker in the practical situation and as a student of health care ethics, with Mr Morris being denied hip replacement surgery?

One response to the question might be this:

- Practically, I could look at access to treatment that may help with Mr Morris's underlying lifestyle difficulties, which are preventing him from having access to surgery (for example, referral to dietetic and smoking cessation services). Success in these areas might ultimately have a positive effect on decisions about access to surgery. We would be on very shaky ethical ground if we omitted to try to help Mr Morris in these ways. Our decision to support treatment denial was based on the belief that it would not truly support his well-being in the sense of capacity for choice and agency, the ground from which positive natural rights and liberties with regard to health care have been constructed. Quite clearly the interventions I have just described *would* do so. Perhaps an important question emerging from this idea is that of whether public health policy is actually robust enough to ensure these interventions.

- Philosophically, we could argue that the decision we have reached (denying expensive surgery but encouraging much less costly lifestyle advice and support) is in accordance with principles of fair distribution of health care resources (Beauchamp and Childress, 2001; Gillon, 1990). But this would only be the case if sufficient resources were allocated through public health policy for this kind of secondary prevention.

It is an empirical fact that health care resources are limited, even in wealthy Western societies (Bradshaw and Bradshaw, 2004; Ham, 2004). It seems to follow, then, that resources should be distributed and allocated according to health **need**, rather than want or whim. But even this statement is not without its problems (Cribb, 2005). What do we mean by 'need'? Whose needs count? How do we decide between the wide ranges of need that are present in our society at any given time?

We can make progress in understanding what we mean by 'need' through distinguishing it from other things, such as 'wants'. Returning to my earlier example of pocket money and flat-screen TVs, we can say that each of these things is a want rather than a need. Both my daughter and I might declare that we need pocket money and televisions, but these claims would be hard to justify. This is because neither the pocket money nor the television will do very much for our basic human rights and freedoms (both negative and positive). Any claim by my daughter that receiving the pocket money will keep her free from poverty, say, or give her the liberty to exercise some crucial aspect of her living would be tenuous. (This is rightly assuming that she has access to other resources apart from the pocket money.) Claims would be still more tenuous, even absurd, in relation to the flat-screen TV. Perhaps I could suggest that having one would fulfil my right to knowledge and understanding by allowing me to watch improving documentary programmes. But then I could fulfil this right in other ways that I have available to me at the moment (libraries, newspapers, radios, my present well-worn television). The point is that we can only talk of something as a 'need' if having it met enables us to an entitled freedom, and not having it met would deny us this freedom (Plant, 2002). The crucial point about the pocket money example is that while earlier I declared that my daughter's pocket money was her natural right (because she had been promised it), this does *not* mean that it is a need and thus of importance in considering entitlement on the basis of distributive justice.

The traditional way in health care of understanding need is related to minimising and, if possible, alleviating ill-health (Cookson and Dolan, 2000). According to this conception, levels of ill-health are the principal determinants of need and it is on these that we should focus when we decide on the use and fair distribution of resources. Within this, there are various ways of understanding the idea of levels of ill-health (and thus need). We can talk of pain and suffering, of immediate threats to life, of 'health opportunities' in the long term to those who are presently sick (or any combination of these). In relation to the latter, for example, it is sometimes claimed that the health needs and entitlements of children suffering from sickness or disability are greater than those who have already lived a long life (Alderson, 1994).

Thinking About...

Reflect on the justifiability (or otherwise) of the idea that children suffering from sickness or disability have greater health need, and thus are more entitled to scarce health care resources, than older people.

Improving Public Welfare: Thinking about Inequalities in Health and Resource Allocation

I have started to address the first in the possible series of questions about need and distributive justice in health care that I outlined above. But the emphasis so far has been on immediate 'medical need' (that is to say, addressing present ill-health in one way or another). This perhaps gives the misleading impression that only illness and disease we are directly experiencing should count in determining need and deciding on how resources should be distributed. If this were the case, then maybe we would not have reached the conclusions that we did about Mr Morris and his access to treatment. After all, he is ill right now and will doubtless secure at least *some* benefit from being treated.

Individual ill-health is extremely important, but it cannot count as the only determinant of health care need simply because other people (apart from the individual concerned) have an interest in how health care resources are allocated and distributed, and with what results. Unless we take an extremely libertarian view of our rights and responsibilities, in addition to the individual we also need to acknowledge the interest of broader society and of the state (the government) in recognising and meeting health care need. We must also understand the importance of the relationship between all three (Cribb, 2005). This leads us to consider two issues that encompass but extend well beyond the question of individual ill-health need:

- The extent to which society and the state should attempt to deal, through the allocation of scarce resources, with **inequalities** in health;
- The degree to which the state should be able to engage in **coercion** of its individual citizens towards more healthful and less risky behaviours.

As I will argue, there is an important connection between these two issues.

Inequalities in health

Although academics and politicians argue about the causes, it is hard to doubt the empirical existence of inequalities in health status. They have been investigated and mapped very carefully since the seminal Black Report in the early 1980s (Townsend et al., 1988; Wilkinson, 1996, 2005). We know that financial resources (or the lack of them), social class, ethnic background and gender all make a difference to how sick we get and how long we live (Wilkinson, 2005). Moreover, we know that the greater the gap between rich and poor in a society, the more likely that dramatic social problems such as crime, violence and other forms of conflict will increase. Thus we are contemplating not only sick individuals but also sick societies (Wilkinson, 2005).

Given this hard-won knowledge and understanding, and its implications for both individuals and the societies in which they live, we expect that the state would want to take action. In particular for our enquiry, we could take the two empirical facts of limited health care resources, on the one hand, and health inequalities, on the other, and argue that relatively more of those resources should be given to those who suffer the most from inequalities. This might lead us towards egalitarian principles for deciding on the allocation of health resources (Cookson and Dolan, 2000).

But while the simple logic of allocating resources according to inequalities in health might seem appealing, the apparent simplicity is complicated by a number of important issues. First, we can say that the broad identification of a particular group as experiencing inequalities is not by itself enough to help reasonable decisions about resource allocation. The evidence is strong that those in lower socio-economic groups suffer worse health and die more quickly than those in higher groupings (Wilkinson, 1996, 2005). But exactly how do we measure lower socio-economic standing? If it is done according to income alone, what exactly divides those who are vulnerable to inequality from those who are not? The conceptualisation and measurement of income inequality has been subject to a great deal of debate (Deacon, 2002). We cannot simply say that everyone earning under £X per week should be privileged with regard to health care resource allocation.

This leads us, second, to the idea that judgements about allocation to address inequalities need to have a finer focus. But here again there is a difficulty. Imagine that we have been able to identify the inhabitants of a particular geographical area as being subject to health inequalities (demographic and epidemiological studies had, say, identified a large out-of-town housing estate as having an especially poor health experience). Assuming, very doubtfully, that inequality is experienced uniformly, we are still left with the problem of who within this supposed uniform group should receive resource benefit.

Example

Within the estate that I have described, on the outskirts of Cardiff, there are two streets. One consists of retirement bungalows for older people and is occupied by a mix of couples and single people, their ages ranging from 60 to 85. In the next street are semi-detached houses occupied mainly by young families. These

(Continued)

(Continued)

two streets are representative of the mixed demography of the estate, where we know that the health experience of almost all is poor.

Funding becomes available to support a community health initiative of some sort. Two proposals are received. One is to support the development of a drop-in and social centre for older people; the other is to fund greater health visitor contact time for work with families. There is not enough money to support both proposals and it cannot be split between two different projects. The question presented to the funding body is which work should it finance, and why.

There is certainly no clear-cut answer here. We might want to take a variation of the so-called 'fair innings' principle and argue that the health visitor work should be funded (Cookson and Dolan, 2000). The older people have already had long lives (or at least longer lives than those of the families). Their 'fair innings' need to be placed against the lives of young parents and children with 'less innings', and resources allocated accordingly. Imagine, though, that within the group of parents there is a significant number who take big 'risks' with their health – smoking, excessive drinking and drug taking. On the other hand, within the group of older people there is a good number who struggle to maintain and preserve their health. Given this addition to the picture, we *might* be prepared to say that the 'opportunity for lifetime health' (Cookson and Dolan, 2000: 328) rests better with abstemious 60 year-olds than with feckless 30 year-old parents. In this case, the decision to fund the work with young families is therefore not so obvious. However, a further variation of the 'lifetime opportunity' argument might suggest that despite the risk-taking of the young parents, there is still more benefit to be had by funding work with them (using the health visiting hours to engage in smoking and drug prevention work, say) than with the older people. But this still yields difficulties:

- By addressing the inequalities present in the first group of young families, we are perpetuating the inequalities in the second group of older people. We may even be creating new inequalities by denying access to health-related services for people who are struggling and doing their best (Cribb, 2005);
- In the context of inequalities in health and the allocation of scarce resources, is there justification in using those resources to support people actively taking 'risks' with their health?

State Coercion and 'Risky' Health Behaviour

We are back in Mr Morris territory, but with one critical difference. Now we can quite clearly see (partly as a result of viewing things through a lens that is to some extent focused on the evidence for inequalities in health) that if we finance Mr Morris's surgery, or support the 'risk-taking' parents, we are potentially at least maintaining or increasing health inequalities. This is simply because by devoting resources to these people, we are denying resources to others, some of whom will be the subject of inequality.

It could be argued in reply that Mr Morris, the parents and many others in similar situations are themselves victims of inequality. It is not their fault that they have become (or are likely to get) sick (Dougherty, 1993). But given that there are also victims of inequality who do not take obvious health risks (the older people on the estate, for example), along with many who have clear 'medical need' in the sense that I discussed it above, why *should* feckless people (disadvantaged or not) have the right to their behaviour? And why *shouldn't* the state take measures to coerce them to more healthful behaviour? After all, won't this result in an improvement to the public welfare in overall terms?

Is there a 'right' to unhealthy behaviour?

The debate over 'rights' to unhealthy behaviour is frequently cast as a moral one (Wikler, 1987). Those who argue that there is no such right resort to a number of obviously ethical arguments, which extend into the territory we have been exploring. An argument from principles of distributive justice claims that, given the scarcity of health care resources, those who behave unhealthily put unfair pressure on those resources by getting sick on their own whim. Moreover, it is argued that if individuals insist on continuing to behave unhealthily, then they forfeit the entitlement to treatment and care provided by the state (Wikler, 1987). In this sense, given what we have said before about 'need' as something that, if met, enables us to an entitled freedom, we cannot properly talk of health risk-takers as possessing need if their present condition is as a result of their own risky behaviour.

A further argument against the 'right' to unhealthy behaviour seems to emerge from the principles of non-maleficence and beneficence. The risk-taker, so it is argued, is exposing himself to the likelihood of harm. We (the state acting on our behalf) have a paternalistic concern for their welfare such that we need to prevent a mistaken 'right' and its exercise (Wikler, 1987).

Q.•Do you think that either (or both) of these arguments *against* the 'right'
•to unhealthy behaviour is acceptable? Justify your response.

There seem to me to be two key difficulties with these arguments against the 'right' to risky health behaviour. First, both (in different ways) presume that exercising it will result in harm for either the individual or the state. The problem is not so much the unhealthy behaviour as what it will lead to (sickness and disease, their unfair burden on the state and harmful effect on the individual). It might be argued that it is hard to untangle the 'right' from its consequences, but this depends on what may be an over-simplistic view of the relationship between cause and effect in disease. While there are strong (sometimes very strong) associative links between certain kinds of lifestyle behaviour and disease (for example, between unhealthy diet and CHD), the links are not causal. Nor is the relationship between intervening to prevent harm (diet modification, say) and that harm (CHD) actually not occurring a causal one (Fitzpatrick, 2001). If I eat poorly, gorging myself on takeaway meals every day, then I'm more likely (quite possibly much more likely) eventually to suffer from CHD, *but it is not a given*. Nor is it given that if I have a blinding revelation, vow never to eat a takeaway again and in future shop only at the whole food store, I will then free myself from the likelihood of CHD. If this is the case, then both distributive and paternalistic arguments against the 'right' to unhealthy behaviour will fail. There is no guarantee, despite my fecklessness, that I will burden the state; nor is it certain that preventing my 'right' out of concern for my welfare will actually result in welfare improvement.

The second difficulty with the presumption against the 'right' to unhealthy behaviour is its fundamental misinterpretation of what is often happening when people engage in unhealthy behaviour. If I eat poorly, say, then this may well not be an exercise of my free will, but rather something that is forced on me – behaviour that has been determined by my social circumstance or my income or my lack of education, or any of a multitude of other things (Lucas and Lloyd, 2005; Tones and Green, 2004). And if behaviour is frequently determined, at least to some extent, we cannot reasonably talk about our 'right' (or lack of 'right') to it at all.

State entitlement to coercion for health

It seems that it is often hard to talk reasonably about the 'right' to risky health behaviour. Where then does this leave the question of the extent to which the state is entitled to intervene coercively to prevent such behaviour and so supposedly improve the public health? While distributive and paternalistic arguments against the 'right' to risky behaviour fail (partly because it is a strange concept in the first place), we might nevertheless feel that an important purpose of state-sponsored health policy and care is prevention of disease, promotion of public health and therefore the improvement of overall public welfare. Engaging with this purpose will almost certainly place us at odds with certain kinds of behaviour, and large numbers of individuals behaving in these ways. But can we actually coerce them into what we ourselves understand to be 'authentic' behaviour?

Certainly, we need to be very wary about strongly coercive practice because, as I have argued, we are talking about behaviour whose consequences are not completely understood and may well be outside individual control. Using an analogy, it would be unfair to imprison a speeding motorist who had some good reason for their fast driving, although we would probably want to apply a more limited sanction or even simply educate him about the dangers of exceeding the speed limit. Equally, though, we do not want to abandon sanctioning or education of speeders because if we did so the rule of the road (and the safety of all its users) would be in jeopardy.

I talked before about the idea that we often accept limits to our health care freedoms, usually without fuss or complaint. This is because, as with the road traffic analogy, our working assumption is often that if our own personal freedom is subject to small limitations, overall freedom and public welfare will be preserved or increased. If I try to keep within the speed limit and am reasonably assured that most other people are attempting to do the same, then I will receive the benefits of a safer road system. If I do what I can to stay healthy and use health care services sensibly and prudently, I will generally benefit. But more than this individual benefit, there is a community benefit from this state of affairs, which relates to, but extends beyond, self-interest. Wikler (1987: 13) calls this 'public health' benefit a 'special kind of good'. We might reasonably suggest that where this public good is in jeopardy because of individual behaviour, consideration should be given to ways of preserving it. These may involve limits to individual action, but not without careful thought about why and what effect any limitation will have.

Conclusion: Health and Welfare – Individual and Public

At the beginning of Chapter 7, describing the territory I hoped to cover in that chapter and this, I raised the issue of both the difference and the connection between 'individual' and 'policy' ethics in health care. I want to return to this now that I have almost reached the end of these chapters.

Questions of individual autonomy have permeated both of the chapters. Regardless of whether our concern is with individual or public welfare, we need to be quite clear that the field of health care is almost always potentially or actually in tension with the autonomy of individuals. For this reason alone, we need to engage in careful construction of what it is to be an individual (a person) and how those (most likely shifting) conceptions of personhood match with our purpose in undertaking health care. However, things are more complicated by the essential need for careful thought about what it is to be a person in society, and as a social person with rights and responsibilities connected to health and health care. As I have said, this dimension of ethical thinking in health care is generally much less well explored than the individual dimension (Cribb, 2005). It seems to be a great deal easier for us to look across to the person we are caring for, to our patient or client, than to look beyond and around at the context that shapes both her and us. Yet this context – the context of government, state, society and community – is central to determining our values, rights, responsibilities and freedoms in health care.

As I have suggested, one way of understanding the difference between health care as individual welfare, on the one hand, and as public welfare, on the other, is through seeing the different spheres as involving different claims, and different relationships based on claims. In general, thoughts about individual welfare involve a fairly narrow set of claims between small numbers of people (often no more than two – the patient and the health care worker, with the former usually having more claims on the latter than the other way around). Public welfare and its improvement, however, involves sets of claims between a much wider range of people, and these claims are often a good deal more 'equal' (between the prudent policy maker and the risk-taking young person, say). Consequently, they may appear much harder to determine. But it is important that we try to do so, and that we work towards connecting up both individual and public welfare claims in our field of interest. I will return to this matter in the final chapter.

Chapter Summary

In this chapter, I have:

- Discussed different conceptions of justice and related these to questions around improving public welfare through health care;
- Explored the implications of the empirical existence of health inequalities for attempts to achieve 'just health care';
- In the context of accounts of justice, rights and freedoms, discussed questions around the limits to unhealthy behaviour and state interventions aimed at improving public health and welfare.

Further Reading

Cribb, A. (2005). *Health and the Good Society: Setting Bioethics in its Social Context*. Oxford: Oxford University Press. This is an extensive discussion of the relationship between bioethics and its social context.

Wilkinson, RG (2005). *The Impact of Inequality*. Abingdon: Routledge. I have tried in this chapter to argue for the empirical existence of inequalities in health playing an important part in ethical deliberations about justice and fairness in health care. This book (along with others by the same author) is a lucid account of why and how inequalities are present in our society, and what effect they have.

9

HEALTH CARE RESEARCH: QUESTIONS OF VALUES AND ETHICS

Learning Outcomes

By the end of this chapter, you should be able to:

o Understand and discuss health care research and research priorities as expressions of value;
o Describe and discuss key ethical issues associated with both the undertaking and the governance of research in health care;
o Describe and discuss some aspects of the relationship between ethics, health care research and global health.

Introduction

Most of my focus so far in this book has been on questions of values and ethics as they relate to health care *practice*. Within this, I have been concerned to demonstrate that values and ethics-related issues permeate all aspects of health care and not simply the dramatic 'life and death' cases that we perhaps most readily think of as the subjects of bioethics. I have very often called this 'ordinary' health care. In trying to demonstrate this, I have been supporting (I hope) my initial claim, made at the very beginning of the first chapter that unless we have a fundamental concern with ethics and values in our health care-related thinking and practice, we can't properly see ourselves as engaged in health care at all. This is just because every aspect of our practice, each kind of contact with patients or clients, has an ethical dimension. Such a dimension will be more or less explicit, but I argue that it will always be present.

In this chapter, I move from thinking about practice to considering **research** and the questions of values and ethics posed within this particular part of the health care domain. I am maintaining, of course, my claim and argument that such questions are fundamental to proper thought about, and involvement in, research. There might be at least two responses to this claim. Somebody might say, 'Yes, of course health care research involves lots of ethical issues. That's why we have ethics committees and the like, to make sure that it's all being done properly.' Someone else could argue, 'Questions of research are so obviously ethical. Think about things like genetic engineering and the development of cutting-edge treatments and interventions. We can't avoid ethics. But these aren't things that I'm personally involved in, so my concern with the ethics of health care research can only ever be limited and second hand.'

Within these two responses are a number of assumptions, which it is part of my purpose in this chapter to examine:

- Health care research is obviously an area for ethical debate;
- Research into new treatments and interventions is the important focus for this debate;
- We are responding to this obvious requirement for debate, and agreement about what is and isn't acceptable, through the mechanisms that are in place for research governance (ethics committees and the like);
- The average health care worker's interest in this area is at best peripheral because she is not actively involved in the kind of 'cutting-edge' health care research that poses 'big' questions of ethics.

I am challenging these assumptions. I want to argue that questions of values and ethics permeate all aspects and kinds of health care research at the levels of both content (what we are researching) and process (how we are going about our research). We should not *simply* be concerned about such things as the ethics of embryo experimentation or trials of a ground-breaking but so far untested drug treatment for cancer, although of course these kinds of areas pose crucial moral questions (Glover, 2006; Kitcher, 1997). My own starting point is the challenge of what I am going to call 'ordinary' research (mirroring my talk of 'ordinary' health care). In doing this, I am following Jon Nixon and Pat Sikes, who, writing specifically about research, say: 'It is not the esoteric, but the customary and the ordinary, that confronts us with the seemingly unanswerable questions' (Nixon and Sikes, 2003).

We are all involved in seeking answers to the customary and the ordinary. Many of us will be involved in what we can reasonably call 'research' in order to try to do so. But those answers may be very hard (or even impossible) to find. In attempting to discover, we are faced with fundamental questions about our methods, and about our relationship with others involved in the research process, including those who have responsibility for its governance.

What is Health Care Research and What is Its Purpose?

In considering the distinction that I am trying to draw between 'cutting-edge' and 'ordinary' health care research, it may be that we come to the view that we *know about* 'cutting-edge' research (through media reports, journal articles, and so on), but actually have *experience of* 'ordinary' research. For example, you might have done, or be undertaking a research project as part of a course of higher or professional education. My aim in this chapter is mainly to explore the ethics of 'ordinary' research, the kind of research that you are perhaps more likely to be involved in. My focus will be largely on thinking about the *process* of 'ordinary' research. In order to do so, I want to generate an example that will help to tease out the ethical difficulty and complexity connected to this kind of research.

Example

Fiona Close is coming to the end of her physiotherapy degree programme. In order to complete the programme, she has to undertake a research project. She has decided that she is most interested in looking at aspects of the social context in which the physiotherapist works; ultimately she wants to practise in the community.

She has recently been involved in a falls prevention scheme for older people in a district of Edinburgh near her university. The community physiotherapist running the scheme organises classes for older people where they can meet each other, receive advice, learn exercise and generally develop confidence that they can move around safely, both at home and in the world outside. The classes are very popular, and Fiona wants to investigate why they are attractive to the people who come, and what effect they have on their confidence.

As Fiona thinks about her potential research project, she starts to consider the question of what health research is, and what purpose it has. Of the many definitions and descriptions she looks at, there is one that seems to be especially helpful: 'At its most general level the conventions of health research can be viewed as work conducted to develop knowledge based on available evidence, following certain rules and procedures' (Saks and Allsop, 2007: 4). This definition and description is helpful almost paradoxically because it is so broad and inclusive. If health research is about the development of knowledge using available evidence, then this legitimates Fiona's enquiry. It is, after all, what she intends to do. She wants to find out from the older people involved in the classes why they find them helpful and what effect they think their involvement has had on them. The idea of the enquiry being legitimated is quite important for Fiona, because what she is doing is rather different from that of some of her peers, who are focusing on the clinical setting. She is also helped by Saks' and Allsops' argument (2007: 7) that health care research is not only about contributing to greater understanding of health, illness and disease, but is also concerned with using this understanding to contribute to policy development in the field. Fiona supposes that if she can develop evidence supporting the usefulness of the falls prevention programme, then it will help in making a case for this kind of work to become more firmly embedded within physiotherapy practice.

But this definition and description also raise important questions. What exactly is to count as 'evidence'? What do we mean when we talk of 'knowledge'? Are some kinds of 'knowledge' and 'evidence' more acceptable than others? What 'rules and procedures' should be followed, and do some have more legitimacy than others?

Health Care Research as the Expression of Values

The distinction between **objectivist and interpretivist paradigms of research**, and the resulting methodologies and methods of the **quantitative researcher**, on the one hand, and the **qualitative researcher**, on the other, are probably familiar to you from courses and texts in research methods. Beginning from the assumption that the world contains objective truths that we can discover, the objectivist uses quantitative methodology and methods (essentially oriented towards measurement) in order to capture these. The interpretivist starts from the position that 'truth' depends on how people understand the world. All we can do is to develop methodology and methods so that we gain some insight into separate understanding and can engage in attempts to interpret this. That is the territory of qualitative research (Holliday, 2002).

These separate positions are not simply statements of fact. They are expressions of value. The objectivist is claiming that value lies in attempts to measure a quantifiable world. The interpretivist is asserting that value rests in recognising and attempting to deal with that which essentially can't be quantified (Holliday, 2002). From these initial expressions of value flow a range of others – the value of particular methods of research, of certain sorts of evidence, and so on.

The 'values difference' between the objectivist and the interpretivist extends, however, well beyond the immediate values related to research and how it is conducted. In health care, differences will be apparent in how they perceive the central values of the field. In Chapter 2, I pointed to separate ways in which the value of health itself might be understood – as an objective state or as subject to interpretation (or possibly a mixture of the two). The debate between the objectivist and the interpretivist health care researcher draws us back to these separate understandings. The objectivist is likely to believe that 'health', as an objective state, can be analysed and measured, and through such measurement it is possible both to determine what needs to be done to improve health and actually undertake this improvement. Meanwhile the interpretivist researcher, attached to the idea of 'health' as something subject to interpretation and not in any sense a fixed entity, will be intent on exploring what it actually seems to mean for people and, given this meaning (or more likely multiple meanings), working out the best kind of response to these different understandings.

Given these separate positions, based on quite different values, we can clearly see that questions of ethics are not simply confined to 'cutting-edge' research. In doing or thinking about research, there will always be a values-related position different from our own. Ethics, as I argued in Chapter 2, is about how we ought to act in order to produce more of what we believe to be valuable. Thus research – both 'cutting-edge' and the 'ordinary' kind more directly relevant to those working in and studying health care – will pose central questions of ethics just because it is fundamentally about values, and centrally involves competition between separate values.

Thinking About...

Reflect on quantitative and qualitative approaches to health care research. Consider the effect that each of these separate approaches might have on the nature and conduct of a particular research activity or project.

Health Care Research: Vulnerability, Power and Control

The pursuit of knowledge and understanding according to particular conceptions of what is valuable very often leads researchers towards patients or clients who, one way or another, provide them with data. The data may be gathered through testing, examination, observation, questionnaire completion and interviews, or in a range of other ways. This encounter and transaction between the researcher and the researched is itself framed by other encounters and transactions, including between the researcher and those involved in the regulation of research – for example, ethics committees. At each level, important ethical questions related to vulnerability, power and control emerge.

The vulnerability of the researched

The clearest vulnerability is perhaps that of the people who are being researched. Fiona Close is acutely aware that she is seeking to work with a group of older people who are either actually or potentially very vulnerable. They may be relatively socially isolated, suffering from age-related physical illnesses, mental health problems, financial hardship, and so on.

Vulnerability (to pain, distress, suffering, and so on) is an essential feature of being properly human. Responding to this vulnerability and its causes is one of the things that makes the acts of those occupations involved in health care moral ones (Edwards, 2001). However, when we are considering the involvement of vulnerable people in research, the nature of the relationship is quite different. While we are caring for somebody, we are responding to needs stemming from their vulnerability; we are trying to *give* them something. When we are researching them, we are not responding to a need; in fact, we could argue that we are *removing* something from them. For example, the older people whom Fiona is researching might give her opinions, views or judgements that they have revealed to nobody else, and perhaps they didn't mean to disclose to her in the first place. On the other hand, granted what Fiona is trying to do, these views could be very helpful in the development of the falls prevention programme and similar schemes elsewhere. The key question is whether this use of a vulnerable group of people to advance knowledge and understanding is ethically acceptable or not (Oliver, 2003).

> Q: How would you justify in an ethical sense the involvement of vulnerable people in health care research? Make a note of your response.

Clearly, either blanket agreement or disagreement to the involvement of vulnerable people in research is an unreasonable position to adopt. Much depends on the individual case – its context, the people involved, what the purpose and nature of the research are, and so on (Oliver, 2003). Moreover, there are two particular dimensions that must be properly thought about and addressed if we are to justify research involving vulnerable people in a particular case:

- There is a need to ensure that those who are being researched give their **consent** to involvement freely. In ensuring this, though, we need to be aware of both the limits and the possibilities of 'informed consent', as I discussed in Chapter 7.
- Because the essential transaction in the research process is one of the researched giving something to the researcher, we must do what we can to promise **confidentiality** to whoever is being researched and what it is that they have given. As Oliver (2003: 83) notes, however, there is a need (as part of the consenting process) to make certain that the person who is being researched knows that the data they generate will be used, and how it will be presented. There may also be circumstances (such as revelations of law-breaking) in which the confidentiality promise cannot be kept. Here, the discussions we have had in Chapters 4 and 5, connected to obligations and principles, might be helpful when thinking about an actual or potential situation.

Careful thought about consent and confidentiality should contribute to the idea that the balance of power between the vulnerable researched and the confident researcher is an important ethical matter, and that it is being addressed.

Example

Fiona often reads in research papers of 'subjects' being recruited for research. In an examination of research methodology literature, she is made aware that how those involved in research are referred to implies much about perceptions of power and control in the research relationship. The researched as a 'subject' might imply a lack of respect for the person who is involved, the sense that he is no more than an instrument that the researcher has to use to get what she wants (Oliver, 2003). If, on the other hand, we talk about research 'participants', this gives a greater sense of equal and active involvement in the work (Nixon et al., 2003). Mindful of debates about vulnerability and the ethics of health care research, Fiona chooses to refer to the older people with whom she is working as participants in her research.

The vulnerability of the researcher: questions of research governance

It may sound odd to talk of 'researcher vulnerability'. After all, as I have discussed, an assumption is often made that in the research relationship the balance of power is held with the researcher (rather than the researched) and it is their ethical obligation to do what they can to make this balance more equal. However, all those engaged in research work in a context and this includes mechanisms for the governance of research. Within these, it is possible to see the researcher as more exposed and vulnerable than we might otherwise think of her as being.

What do we mean when we talk of 'governance'? :

> Governance is a term used to refer to the systems by which organisations govern themselves or are governed – how the conduct of an organisation is conducted. (Boden, 2004: 4)

The notions of 'government' and 'conduct' imply that there are certain standards that must be reached and maintained in order for conduct to be acceptable. Thus governance itself has an important ethical dimension (Boden, 2004). Research governance is the government and regulation of conduct with regard to research taking place within or from an organisation. In the health care context, this is often the NHS, or it may be the organisation (such as a university) from which the researcher is working.

When we think of how research in or involving the NHS and universities is regulated and conducted, we perhaps most frequently think of ethics committees. For the NHS, it is a requirement that independent review of any proposed research involving patients or staff (among others) is obtained from a Local Research Ethics Committee (LREC) (Central Office for Research Ethics Committees, 2001). LRECs are made up of a number of lay and professional members, whose key purpose is to try to examine the proposed research – its likely benefits, potential problems, and so on – from the point of view of the 'ordinary person' (Alderson, 2007: 291).

Example

Because Fiona's research involves NHS patients, she has to submit an application for ethical approval to her LREC. She is asked to attend the meeting at which the application will be discussed. She arrives early and while waiting to go in chats to another applicant, who is undertaking research on the potential benefit of electrical stimulation accompanying exercise in stroke rehabilitation. He tells Fiona that his colleague's application is also being discussed this evening. This colleague is researching the effect of polyunsaturated fatty acids and monosaturated fats on digestion during rest and exercise. Fiona thinks about her own work and the simple asking of questions to a group of older people. With some trepidation, she enters the committee room where the members of the LREC, mostly men in suits together with a couple of women in smart dresses, sit waiting for her. After some preliminaries, one of the suited men says to her, 'I'm not sure what you're trying to do here. It seems as if you're just asking a few questions. Is that right?'

There is a little caricature in my example now, but not too much. It is certainly true, as Fiona is experiencing, that LRECs (along with other parts of the machinery of NHS governance) are sources of power and arenas in which struggles for power take place (Alderson, 2007). They have the power to refuse Fiona permission to undertake her research, or to require her to amend what she is doing. Moreover, it may be that in the exercise of this power, members of the committee are subscribing to certain values, or conceptions of values, that are not necessarily shared by Fiona. One of the frequently voiced criticisms of LRECs is that they are biased against social science research in general, and qualitative methods in particular (Alderson, 2007). If we return to our discussion earlier in this chapter about the assumptions of the objectivist and the interpretivist with regard to the nature of knowledge in health care, we can perhaps say that members of Fiona's LREC might well see 'health' in a different way from her. For them, 'health' is maybe seen as quantifiable – the absence of disease, as according to the medical model. Perhaps this is what lies behind the particular member's comment in this interlude during the evening where the focus is removed for a while from narrow, clinical research. (Think of the other research that is being reviewed during the evening and how this work might attempt conceptually to frame 'health'.) At the same time, Fiona is struggling to develop an understanding of health that depends heavily on how individuals are situated in their social context. It is quite easy to see how the LREC forms an arena for a power struggle, although we could reasonably argue that the balance, by virtue of what the committee can do and decide, is firmly on its side. We may well be inclined to see Fiona, her assumptions, beliefs and values as highly vulnerable in this context, and to agree with Boden that:

> Corporate governance [here in the cause of research ethics] is just part of a system of interlocking regimes of practice that shape our thinking and lead to the exercise of power in contemporary societies. (Boden, 2004: 23)

Thinking About...

Reflect on this conception of research ethics governance and its implications for research practice.

'Evidence' and research hierarchies

Issues of power and control connected to research ethics do not, however, simply end in the LREC committee room, in exchanges between their members and applicants, and in decisions that are made there. The wider health care arena is essentially characterised by beliefs about what counts as 'evidence' for its interventions and treatments, and about what kind of research produces acceptable evidence. In Chapter 5, I discussed the place of the randomised controlled trial (RCT) as the 'gold standard' in health care and medical research (Tones and Green, 2004). In the context of this discussion on the ethics of health care research, we can now frame the RCT, and new knowledge and understanding generated through RCT-based research, as being at the pinnacle of a hierarchy of evidence. Further down the hierarchy are such things as meta-analyses, systematic reviews of effectiveness, literature reviews, and so on (Tones and Green, 2004). But it is the RCT and its outcomes that provide the soundest 'evidence' from the research base to inform decisions about practice.

This belief is one of the mainstays of the so-called evidence-based medicine (EBM) movement. The ideas that provided the impetus to the movement developed from the early 1970s, especially the work of Cochrane, who argued that health care treatments should be based on sound evidence that they actually *worked* (Worrall, 2007). This may sound obvious, but Cochrane was able to present a case showing that many treatments and interventions in medicine and health care were based on criteria other than effectiveness and efficacy, and were often undertaken simply because this was what had always been done. (Perhaps the most famous example he provided was that of the insertion of grommets for glue ear in childhood.)

My purpose is certainly not to argue against the importance of medicine and health care working from a strong base of evidence. As John Worrall says, the idea that medical science and medical practice should be based on evidence is 'surely a "no- brainer"' (Worrall, 2007: 1). It would be more than perverse to try to argue that evidence shouldn't enter our heads when we think about what to do in health care. However, I do want to raise two closely linked issues related to EBM (and evidence-based health care (EBHC) in general) that are important in discussion on the ethics of research:

- The danger of distorting the relationship between health care knowledge and how it is acquired (epistemology) and health care ethics;
- The risk of 'evidence' taking priority over all other contributors to decisions about how we should frame practice and what it should be based upon.

EBM and EBHC for a long time seemed to possess the quality of evangelical movements. Their ideas, and the language in which they were expressed, were unequivocal. There was a requirement to *believe*, or for the EBM-ers to convert someone to belief. Members of the movements wished to de-emphasise intuition as a component of practice decision-making, and to question the use of unsystematic clinical expertise in what was being done (Worrall, 2007). While this evangelism has been tempered over time, there are still certain fundamental beliefs to which EBM and EBHC cling. One of these is that RCTs carry greater weight in terms of what counts as knowledge than other methods of discovery. Despite the tempering that has taken place, this is still a powerful message because what it essentially implies is the following. If we believe that health care is about improving the lives of individuals, communities and populations, and if we also believe that effective interventions are needed to do this, then we must place most faith in the research method that is most likely to show us what interventions are indeed effective (that is to say, the RCT). But this implication is dangerous because, as I have tried to argue throughout this book, relying on one moral imperative alone (the production of benefit) will not allow us to deal with the individual and social complexity of ethical decision-making. We need to account for, and think about, much more. Simply to say that objective knowledge equals good decisions (which is not so far off the claims of the EBM-ers) is very risky indeed.

If we accept the complexity of ethical decision-making, we also have to allow that we use multiple sources to understand what is going on and what needs to be done. So we need to allow that there will be other contributors to the decisions we make, and these will include such things as intuition and 'unsystematically' developed clinical expertise, the kinds of things that those wedded to EBM and EBHC have traditionally played down. Indeed, we could reasonably argue about what is meant by 'unsystematic'. If it is simply another word for 'irrational', then there is a need to remind ourselves that rational thinking is only one aspect of a properly reflective approach to what we do in health care, and that it needs to be accompanied by attempts to reconcile and account for our emotions and feelings as well (Tate and Sills, 2004).

Thinking About...

Consider the extent to which the principles and beliefs of EBM and EBHC affect your views on what kind of research should be undertaken in health care, and how it should be used and applied in practice.

Research and Global Health

Debates about the evidence base for medicine and health care are perhaps a luxury that only health care workers and researchers in the affluent countries of the West can afford to have. I want briefly to focus on the issue of research ethics in the context of **global health**.

The existence of profound inequalities in health between the First and the Third Worlds is well documented. It extends beyond the simple but highly alarming facts of morbidity, mortality and disease incidence and prevalence to very deep-seated structural problems related to international trade, wealth and transnational organisations (Macdonald, 2006). Given this, issues of ethics in the context of international research and global health are pressing and urgent. The Nuffield Council on Bioethics has framed the problem in this way:

> Many people in the developing world suffer from poor health and reduced life expectancy. The role of research that contributes to the development of appropriate treatments and disease prevention measures is vital. However, lack of resources and weak infrastructure mean that many researchers in developing countries have very limited capacity to conduct their own clinical research. They therefore undertake research in partnership with groups from developed countries. A sound ethical framework is a crucial safeguard to avoid possible exploitation of research participants in these circumstances. (Nuffield Council on Bioethics, 2005: xiii)

Although there is good reason and empirical evidence to doubt the ethics of First World commitment to Third World health care research (see, for example,

Macdonald (2006)), my brief focus and argument here is on the need (and perhaps the difficulty) of understanding and framing research, its underpinning motivations and ethics in quite different ways in poorer countries. To begin with, familiar concepts, such as consent to participation in research, may require careful thought. There is a need to take account of cultural differences. Roles associated with gender may be much more traditional and demand different ways of understanding how consent is sought and gained. Alternative conceptions of community might also prompt rethinking with regard to issues such as consent and standards of care during research. Crucially, if the First World is serious about moving towards redressing the balance in terms of power and understanding, a great deal of emphasis must be placed on the empowerment of people and communities involved in research. Ensuring their participation and arranging things so that there is maximum chance of sustainability once outside involvement in the research has ended also seem very important. Finally, there is a need to think about reorientation of the research agenda away from the 'high tech' and towards areas such as public health and primary care, where a great deal more difference is likely to be made to the lives of many more people living in poorer countries (Benatar and Singer, 2000; Nuffield Council on Bioethics, 2005).

Thinking About...

Consider what might be included on your own checklist of what it is important to ensure in order that health care research in developing countries is planned and conducted ethically.

Conclusion: the Enduring Connection between Ethics and Research in Health Care

Towards the beginning of this chapter, I introduced the example of Fiona Close and her particular concerns about the progress of the qualitative research project that she was planning to undertake. Near its end I have raised issues related to the connection between ethics, research and global health. The wide sweep of potential interest related to research ethics – from the particular to the global – is one representation of the inevitable, crucial and enduring connection between research and questions of values and ethics.

As I have argued, the connection is such because our research choices (about both what we choose to investigate and how we decide to do so) are embedded in values. As a result of this, we are faced with questions of ethics – why it is that we value what we do and how it might be possible to produce more of what we understand to be valuable. In this respect, health care *research* is no different from health care *practice*, for these are the kinds of questions that have run right the way through this book.

What *is* different, I have argued, is the nature of our response to issues of health care research ethics. In the first place, there is perhaps a tendency for us to confine the ethical problematic in research to the high technology of genetics, advanced treatments, and so on. In contrast, although many might see the ethical dilemmas of practice as being represented in these kinds of 'large' questions, it is also possible to draw on an increasing range of resources (as I have tried to do in this book) that locate questions of ethics firmly in the everyday of 'ordinary' health care. Second, efforts at 'governmentality' (to adopt a term from Foucault) (Boden, 2004: 8) seem much more focused in relation to research ethics than the ethics of practice. Of course, we can point to pervading professional structures and things like codes of conduct that are clearly attempting to ensure ethical governance of health care practice. However, every time in our practice that we approach a patient, we do not have to clear hurdles of 'ethical approval', whereas this is (or should be) always the case when we seek patient participation in research.

However, the difficulty with the ever-present governance of research ethics, as I have argued, is that in paying close attention to what *we* (as actual or potential researchers) are doing, it draws attention away from the substantial difficulties with the process of governance itself. Problems of power, vulnerability and control exist within systems for the regulation and conduct of research. It is essential that they are subject to as much thought and scrutiny as the actual relationship between the researcher and the researched that the systems have ostensibly been set up to monitor and regulate.

Chapter Summary

In this chapter, I have:

- Argued for the pervasiveness of questions of values and ethics within health care research, whatever its nature;
- Discussed issues of power, vulnerability and control and their central importance within both individual research and structures for the governance of research ethics;
- Argued that global research ethics poses a particular challenge, at least partly as a result of the existence of profound inequalities between nations.

Further Reading

Nuffield Council on Bioethics (2005). *The Ethics of Research Related to Health Care in Developing Countries*. London: Nuffield Council on Bioethics. This discussion paper raises many interesting issues related to the ethics of health care research in the Third World.

Oliver, P (2003). *The Student's Guide to Research Ethics*. Maidenhead: Open University Press. Oliver provides a 'how to' guide on research ethics, as well as discussion of overarching issues. The focus is on research generally, rather than health care research particularly.

10

FRAMEWORKS FOR FURTHER THINKING

Learning Outcomes

By the end of this chapter, you should be able to:

○ Identify, describe and discuss a range of areas for further thinking and debate related to issues of values and ethics in the health care context;
○ Identify processes and resources that might help with your further thought.

Introduction

I have two main purposes in this final chapter. First, I want to review progress through the book, focusing especially on key areas where there seems to be particular scope for further thinking and discussion. Second, I want to suggest some ways in which you might actually go about engaging in further thinking and debate, and some resources that might be helpful to you in doing so.

Further thinking about values and ethics in the health care context is certainly not compulsory! It may be that you have reached the end of this book, or have used it as you wish, and the last thing you want to do is to think more about ethics and values. Perhaps you have used this book to support your learning on a particular course and now the course has ended you are moving on to something else. The desires to move on or to abandon formal thought about values and ethics are quite understandable. However, I hope that any abandonment will not be complete, given the central claim and theme of this book – that unless we have a concern with values and ethics, we can't properly see ourselves as engaging in health care at all, given the field's purposes, nature and practices.

The suggestions I am about to make, in terms of both areas for further thought and processes to support your doing so, are not exclusive. The study of values and ethics poses endless questions of interest; application to the practical health care context serves to make or reinforce those questions as ones that are crucially important and engaging. An important theme of the book has been that this is the case not only with regard to dramatic 'life and death' health care, but also the ordinary and everyday practices with which the vast majority of health care workers are mainly involved. I hope by now you will be in a position where you recognise that your own practice (or potential practice) in health care is very fertile ground for values and ethics-related exploration.

Thinking About...

Each chapter of this book, and especially many of the 'Thinking About' and 'Q' features, have encouraged you to reflect on your values as a worker, or potential worker, in health care, as well as how you might think or feel about, and react to, contexts and situations in which issues of ethics emerge. Review your responses to these and consider the picture they should have built up of health care as a values and ethics-laden context, and of yourself within this.

Areas for Further Thinking and Debate

I want to begin by considering possible areas for further thinking that have emerged as a result of the discussions in this book. To do so, I'm going to return to the three case studies that we started out with in Chapter 1: Dr Irwin and Mrs Murphy; childhood obesity; and Joe, the 11 year-old who suffers from autism and severe developmental delay. My intention is to use the book's discussions to pose a 'new' set of questions about the cases. These questions certainly do not lead to answers to the major values and ethics-related uncertainties that the three studies represent. As I have tried to argue through the book, 'answers' (in the sense of complete and undisputable verdicts about what should be done, how we should react, and why) do not exist. What it is possible to achieve, though, through thought, reflection and discussion, is a greater understanding of the nature of difficulties and how it might be possible to approach them. I hope that these questions serve to extend our thinking about the three cases that we began with, as well as your own thought about your actual or potential practice as you move on from this book.

Question 1: What health care-related values do you hold, and why do you hold these?

We began our discussion about the nature of values in health care in Chapter 2. A central part of my argument then was that the experience of becoming and being a health care worker was fundamental in the formation of values. This experience helped to frame beliefs about the nature of the value of health itself and the value of particular kinds of health care approaches. For example, despite prolonged encounters with other ways of understanding the nature of the value of health, the deeply embedded character of professional values might still incline us towards seeing it as 'absence of disease', and the value of health care as lying in the treatment and care it offers to ameliorate sickness and ill-health. This focus on values, and especially the acquisition of values through professional training and experience, in fact helps us better to understand what is happening in each of the case studies. In all three, what we are struggling with are conceptions of the value of life and living. As I have argued through many of the chapters of this book, the value of life is intimately connected with further values, including the values of health and of well-being. The cases of Dr Irwin and Mrs Murphy, childhood obesity and Joe, the boy with autism, all allow for the possibility of quite different understandings of what health (and well-being) actually are – and of what is the nature of the values of health and health care. Health care could be the use of technology and skills to retain life as long as possible *or* it could be the seeking of release from pain and peaceful death (Dr Irwin and Mrs Murphy). Health might be the absence of disease, achieved through strict regimens of behaviour *or* it could be throwing all caution to the wind and having a good time (debates about obesity). Again, health might involve the search for meaning in your own life *or* the ascription of meaning to the lives of others (the case of Joe).

The point is not that we have to adopt any or all of these understandings of the value of health and health care. Rather, it is to recognise that different and potentially incompatible understandings are possible and that what we ourselves believe to be the nature of the value is likely to differ from the beliefs of others. Moreover, if we are (or are in the process of becoming) professionals working in health care, we are likely to be subject to particular influences on our understanding. These influences will heavily frame our view of the case studies, and what it would be best to do in order to preserve values according to our beliefs about what they entail.

Question 2: How are our values and the ethical positions we hold shaped by the pluralist society in which we live?

Throughout this book, we have encountered a challenge to the normative ethical theories and positions of Western, post-Enlightenment liberal society. The challenge is often implicit but it is crucial. It emerges from the fact that we no longer live in a society where liberal values (the primacy of the individual, the essential importance of autonomy, and so on) are necessarily shared. Our society is pluralist, shaped by different cultures and religions, with differences in ideology and values emerging as a result. As I discussed in Chapter 5, even theories of bioethics (such as the four principles), which explicitly set out to try to be acceptable to all, can be challenged. Such things as the fundamental importance of community or of the patriarch may replace, for some, a traditional set of liberal values.

I don't want to suggest that we can't move towards reconciling separate cultural traditions and all they mean for social organisation. What I do want to claim, though, is that if we are to engage in careful thinking about health care ethics, we have to consider particularly what the fact of our living in a pluralist society might mean for our ethical reasoning and decision-making.

For example, what could the fact of pluralism mean for our three case studies? We might suggest that for Dr Irwin and Mrs Murphy, we need to balance views about the importance of individual autonomy with others that emphasise the significance to particular communities of our reasoning and decisions. This case symbolises questions of life and death, and our reactions to it are highly dependent on our cultural background (quite apart from what the law governing our society actually says can and cannot be allowed). But the other case studies are equally symbolic. With regard to childhood obesity, an emphasis on community, for example, might completely change our views on what should be done; it could be argued that obesity drains our community resources and therefore strong preventative action is required irrespective of the effect on personal autonomy. As for Joe, differences emerging from pluralism seem to heighten debates about the nature of the 'worthwhile life' that his case seems to represent. We could argue, for example, that the common good supporting lives such as Joe's is what makes his (and every other) life important, regardless of individual capacity and autonomy.

Once again, in each of the cases, we can see that posing this kind of question is likely to change or reshape the ethical position from which we began.

Question 3: What is the relationship between the individual and her own moral perspectives, and the social context within which all issues of ethics are framed?

This question is connected to the previous one, but extends beyond it. We need to think not only about the pluralism of values, but also about the plurality of social contexts and situations in which values are developed and decisions are made. When I come to a decision about what to do or how to act, it can only very partly be understood as an individual action. It is heavily framed by my social situation. When I decide to go out to the pub, or not to enrol on an evening class, or buy the cheap brands at the supermarket, my social context and situation plays a huge part – my education, employment, income, support network, and so on.

As I have argued, the social context in which issues of ethics develop has often been neglected in any attempts to understand what is going on and what should be done. The focus instead has been on action at the individual level. Of course, this is critically important, but it needs to be connected to attention towards the broader social context. Taking the three case studies again, we can see the effect that this wider spotlight will have on our deliberations. Her background, her support networks, her social history as a health care patient, and so on will all frame Mrs Murphy and her actions with Dr Irwin. Equally, placing childhood obesity in the social context in which the 'problem' has developed will help our understanding. We might see it as related to questions of inequality, or the medicalisation of ordinary life. Again, seeing Joe as a social being rather than a 'medical difficulty' is likely to alter our attitudes towards his case.

These different 'takes' on the cases we began with, inspired by thoughts about their social context, are certainly not compulsory. But if we don't consider them, we seem to be missing out on so much that could help our ethical understanding.

Question 4: How do we prepare ourselves for dealing with the extraordinariness of ordinary situations?

I have tried to keep the balance and focus of this book firmly on the ethics of 'ordinary' health care. This is because the everyday situations implied in my use of the term are the ones that you are most likely as a health care worker to encounter – advising a patient about their lifestyle, dealing with the effects of a smoking ban, supporting an elderly person faced with the possibility of no longer living in their own home, and so on. But as I hope I have demonstrated, within each of these kinds of ordinary situations is an extraordinariness that compels our attention and presents us with very real dilemmas – no less real than the 'life and death' that is often the concern of bioethics. The question, then, is one of how we prepare ourselves for dealing with the constant presence of an ethical dimension in our 'ordinary' health care lives.

Among the ways that we can prepare ourselves, I want to refer back to two particular discussions in earlier chapters – about obligations on the one hand, and virtues on the other. We can (admittedly rather artificially) create two different kinds of health care workers concerned with ethics. One believes that he is guided by obligations, already framed in the code of conduct that drives his profession and his work. The other believes that the responsibility for deciding what to do lies largely with her and she needs to develop this moral capacity from within. These two workers would have quite different ways of preparing themselves for the challenges of practice. For the first, it would be about developing familiarity with his obligations; for the second, her concern would be with developing moral capacity through observation, vicarious learning, and so on.

What we might want to suggest, as I did earlier, is that neither obligations nor virtues on their own provide us with sufficient resources to deal with the 'extraordinariness of the ordinary'. We need to know both what is required of us, and what we require of ourselves. We need to engage in each kind of preparation. This view is perhaps different from the one that we started out with when we first came across the three case studies in Chapter 1. We may have believed at this point that what counted was being aware of 'set in stone' theories and positions, which would provide us with definitive guidance. This, I have claimed and argued, is not so. Now we begin to see the cases and how we think about them in a different light. We should not be approaching Dr Irwin and Mrs Murphy, the issue of childhood obesity and 11 year-old Joe simply as instances of rules application. Rather, we should be using the rules that we know are out there to inform (along with other things such as experience, intuition and independent thought) our ethical awareness of the situations. The difference with this approach is that we are now not coming to each situation with the question, 'What should be done?' Instead, our starting point is, 'I have thought before about these kinds of things. I have learnt from others. I have, and am developing, my ethical personality. Therefore I am ready to face the challenge, with the benefit of experience, of this new situation.' This conveys, as it should, a much greater sense of empowerment in dealing with the ethical issues that face us daily in the practice of health care that is 'extraordinary in its ordinariness'.

Thinking About...

Consider these four questions for yourself, in relation to either the case studies (as I have done) or to an ethical situation in your own practice or potential practice.

Processes and Resources for Further Thinking

The intention of the questions I have just posed is to provide a framework, based on the discussions within this book, for the extension of your thinking about ethical issues in health care practice. These are certainly not the only questions that could be asked in order to support the development of thinking. It is possible to imagine further questions, either different from those that I have set out or in some way related to them. For example, there could be a sub-set of questions connected to my own final one about preparation for dealing with the 'extraordinary of the ordinary' in health care, questions on the use and limits of codifying ethics, problems connected with the idea of learning to be virtuous, and so on.

If we take it seriously, however, the task of asking questions requires direction and support. Some of this might be available from other people, but you may have to generate much by yourself. What I want to do now is to set out particularly how you might go about further exploration and questioning. My focus will be two-fold. The first is on the processes that might be helpful in ethical exploration – the ways in which you might continue to expose tensions, demonstrate difficulties and move towards greater understanding. The second is on the resources that might help you in these tasks.

Further thinking: processes

Perhaps talk about setting out ways of engaging in processes that will lead to further thinking is a bit misleading because my main intention is actually to emphasise (or re-emphasise) some of the processes that I have tried to develop in this book. It would be rather odd if I were to write a book about values and ethics in the health care context in a certain way and then suggest at its end that the reader should go off and think about things in a completely different way! I hope that the routes by which I have approached the issues raised in this book have led to some illumination, and that considering how this has been arrived at might provide the basis of a model for moving on in thought and reflection. Perhaps more importantly, what I have tried to do in this book is to model philosophical-ethical ways of arguing and thinking. Once again, it would seem more than a bit odd to write a book about health care values and ethics without trying to engage in the processes that ethical thinkers use themselves. So this book that you are reading about ethical thinking is modelled on the processes of ethics, which I am now asking you to consider as ways of extending your own thought. My hope is that there will then be symmetry between your approach and mine, and between these and the work of others, which has provided guidance for us through this present text. (In saying this, I'm not suggesting that we always have to slavishly follow others' ways of thinking. Rather I'm claiming that there is very often value in learning from a discipline's traditions and ways of working (Duncan, 2007).)

The importance of dialogue

The roots of philosophy as a discipline (and therefore of ethics) lie in **dialogue**. The Ancients, beginning with Socrates, generally believed that philosophical enquiry was best conducted through the interplay of opinions and co-operative enquiry (Lacey, 1976: 51). This idea of logical argument or dialogue as an engine that drives discovery was termed **dialectics** – literally a 'method of conversation or debate' (Lacey, 1976: 51) – and the word is still understood in this way today. However, there is another modern meaning of dialectic, which is that it is the identification of a contradictory process (Bonnett, 2001). An idea (thesis) is opposed by another idea (anti-thesis) and a synthesis of the contradiction eventually emerges. In its representation and disentanglement of thesis and anti-thesis, the synthesis should demonstrate greater understanding than existed at the point of the original thesis.

Although dialectic has these two different meanings of logical debate and contradictory process, I take them both (actually or potentially) to involve dialogue. And it is dialogue, the interplay of ideas in one way or another, which is so important to the development of thinking around values and ethics in health care. Dialogue is important because:

- It allows for the demonstration of different ideas;
- It allows for difficulties and possibilities within ideas to be shared;
- As a result of this, it allows us to reach new understanding (we may either move to a new position or feel strengthened in the one that we have already adopted).

Dialogue should, in the Socratic tradition, be genuinely co-operative if we are to gain the greatest benefits from it. If it is conducted with an eye to conflict or points scoring, the learning to be gained from it will be limited. The limits will be imposed because we will be looking to win, rather than to understand.

One of the difficulties in emphasising the importance of dialogue in developing further thinking on values and ethics is that you may be unclear about how to develop dialogic processes, or who to have dialogue with. I will consider this difficulty further in my discussion of resources to aid further thinking.

The worth of examples

Philosophers rely heavily on examples to underpin, illustrate and develop their arguments. They are not unique in doing so; many other academic disciplines also use examples to extend their argument and debate (or they use closely associated things, such as case studies, and so on). However, examples have a particularly important place in philosophy, and therefore ethics. As we discussed in Chapter 4, the arguments of ethics are often *a priori*; they are constructed independently of experience. The utilitarian, say, does not go out to question 5,000 people and come back with the verdict that the vast majority of those surveyed believe that NHS finances should be allocated according to the greatest happiness principle. Her argument depends on reason alone and not empiricism. However, we recognised in our discussion the difficulty of constructing a purely *a priori* argument. There has to be some reference to things as they are, or as they might be, in order to ground the argument. Given the philosopher generally has no wish to rely on fieldwork to support his argument, it follows that the examples grounding them need to be as effective and as useful as possible.

In considering how you might extend your ethical thinking, the importance of examples in philosophical-ethical argument suggests two things:

- It is essential to assess the worth of others' examples (say, writers whom you are reading) in order to come to conclusions about the worth of their argument as a whole;
- It is also crucial to think very carefully about the value of any examples you might generate yourself in order to justify the direction and content of your thinking.

Examples can illuminate and support. They can help in the building of strong grounds for argument or they can cloud issues and weaken cases. Recognising and developing good examples is a highly useful skill to develop as you move forward in your health care-related ethical thinking.

The importance of both critical analysis and critical reflection

Critical analysis is the process of attempting to understand the nature and meaning of something (for example a concept or theory) by examining it in detail (Tate, 2004). **Critical reflection** is the process of thinking about thinking and experiences in a way that enables somebody to learn from what they have encountered (Marshall and Rowland, 1998). Critical analysis largely involves cognition (thinking), while critical reflection extends beyond cognition alone to embrace consideration of feelings, emotions and attitudes (Tate, 2004). It must do so simply because true learning involves not only rational cognition but also affection (feeling, and so on). I argue that if we wish to extend our thinking about values and ethics in health care, we need to develop our capacity for both analysis and reflection.

This may sound rather surprising – surely philosophy and ethics are above all else about logic and rationality? And if this is so, shouldn't analytic thinking alone be the key to progress? Certainly, critical analysis is important. In order to understand a concept (for example, 'health'), careful examination through breaking it down into its constituent parts is crucial. This is the kind of process that I have attempted throughout this book, and I have also encouraged you as the reader to engage in it. However, as I have discussed in Chapter 2 and elsewhere, the acquisition of values, and therefore of particular ethical positions, is not a wholly rational process. We acquire these things through our personal and professional experience. This involves our whole selves – the emotional and social, as well as the rational. Developing capacity for critical reflection as well as critical analysis will help us:

- Understand more fully why we adopt the values and ethics-related positions that we do;
- Understand more fully why others adopt their own positions, which may or may not be different from ours.

Further thinking: resources

Each of the processes that I have described as being likely to support further understanding and debate is not necessarily easy to engage with. There is a need for help and support. I want now to offer some brief pointers towards resources that might be of use to you.

Yourself and your colleagues

Perhaps it sounds blindingly obvious, but it is often strangely overlooked that you and the people you work or study with are your primary resource for further thinking about values and ethics in health care. You (and hopefully your colleagues) are actively thinking about the questions and issues we have been discussing. You have been reading about them. You have (or at least are likely to have) experiences that will allow you to analyse and reflect on problems within practice. If you are lucky, you will have colleagues from both within and outside your own profession or occupation who will be doing similar things. Nevertheless, it would be wrong-headed to deny that there might well be difficulties in making the most of yourself and your colleagues.

> Q: What difficulties might exist in using yourself and/or your colleagues as resources for further thinking and debate? List these.

Your list might have included things such as lack of time, interest, opportunity and commitment. Some or all of these (and others) might apply equally to you and your colleagues. Or they might apply to one or other of you. It is worth spending some further time working out exactly where the difficulty lies and what, if anything, can be done to overcome the problem. It is also worth establishing exactly why you want to engage in further thinking and debate. What is its purpose and benefit? As I said at the beginning of this chapter, further thinking is not compulsory. Equally, it might be difficult for you at this particular time, for any number of reasons. If this is so, then you might find it easier to move on. Such moving on might be for good, or it might be just for now. My own hope is that moving on for you will be temporary rather than permanent. I hope that to some degree my argument in this book for the fundamental importance of values and ethics in health care has been convincing. But whether and for how long you decide to move on, you will be doing so for your own reasons, and these will be important.

The use of 'everyday' resources

Questions of values and ethics, as I have argued, are ever-present in our lives. Yet one of the arguments often made for difficulties in teaching ethics to those in occupational or professional training (who may well be quite young) is that they do not have enough experience to use as help in reasoning and the formation of judgements (Halper, 2003). Drawing together this view with that of the ever-present nature of values and ethics supplies us with clues as to how we might move forward in gathering 'experience'.

Values and ethics as 'everyday' means that questions related to them are not confined to rare professional experience. We can use our ordinary experience to help our reasoning. More particularly, if we are anxious about this use, or need to have time to engage in careful analysis, we can use the vicarious experience of ethical dilemmas gained through media. In television, films and books, we are frequently presented with characters debating ethical situations and choices. (In fact, it could be argued that this is the defining feature of good story and narrative.) They will obviously not all be health care workers presented with the kinds of questions that you face, but with imagination and sympathy the experiences we watch or read about can be used vicariously. Halper (2003), for example, discusses the use of Woody Allen's film, *Crimes and Misdemeanours* to prompt ethical debate. Macnaughton (2007) analyses Ian McEwan's novel, *Saturday*, in a search for understanding of what it means to be a 'good doctor'. It is worth spending time thinking about both the actual and vicarious 'everyday' experience that we all have in which questions of values and ethics are present, and how we can use them for our own learning.

> ### Thinking About...
>
> Identify and reflect on a novel, film or other media resource that you think could be a useful learning and teaching resource for the extension of thinking related to values and ethics.

E-resources

It is probably easier now than it has ever been to find and use the work of both contemporary and past philosophers. It is possible (through 'blogs') to read philosophers' thoughts as they emerge, and even to participate in virtual philosophical discussion. Without abandoning the criteria of selection and critical judgement that we would use when working out what to read and use in the 'real' world, the 'virtual' world of the Internet can be very useful in exploring ethical themes and arguments, and helping to develop your further thought.

While what is available through the Internet is fluid and changing, which of course is one of the difficulties with the medium, a reliable guide is provided by Intute, a free online web reference service provided by a network of universities in the United Kingdom (www.intute.ac.uk/artsandhumanities/philosophy). The Higher Education Academy Health Sciences and Practice Subject Centre (www.health.heacademy.ac.uk) has an interest in developing teaching and learning related to ethical thinking in health care practice, especially as they are connected to collaborative and interprofessional learning.

Conclusion: A Final Word

In this chapter, I have sketched out some ways of extending thinking on values and ethics in the health care context, both in terms of processes that can be developed and resources that can be used in supporting further work. But this can only be a sketch, suggestive of a way forward. It certainly can't be prescriptive. Any prescription is impossible because, as I hope this book has demonstrated, the ways of thinking about ethics are complex and contested, as are any conclusions that we might be likely to reach. The only firm conclusion that might be possible in thought about values and ethics in health care is that the terrain to be explored is risky and uncertain.

In my view, this should not stop us from exploration. Indeed, it is the very difficulty that seems to make that exploration both exciting and worthwhile. I hope that what you have read, and what you have thought about as a result of reading, has played a part in convincing you of that. The next steps, if you choose to take any, are up to you.

Chapter Summary

In this chapter, I have:

- Outlined and discussed a range of areas, represented by questions, that will help you towards further thinking about values, ethics and health care;
- Described and discussed processes and resources that might support further exploration of the field.

Further Reading

Both of these books may help you especially with the processes of developing argument and reflecting on your responses to the actions, arguments and positions of others. I have personally found both very helpful, but of course there are many others that might be equally of use to you:

Bonnett, A (2001). *How to Argue*. Harlow: Pearson Education.

Warburton, N (2007). *Thinking from A to Z* (Third Edition). Abingdon: Routledge.

REFERENCES

Alderson, P (1994). What right to health care? *Healthmatters*, 20, 18–19.

Alderson, P (2007). Governance and ethics in health research. In Saks, M and J Allsop (eds), *Researching Health*. London: Sage, 283–300.

Armstrong, D (1983). *Political Anatomy of the Body*. Cambridge: Cambridge University Press.

Armstrong, D (1993). From clinical gaze to regime of total health. In Beattie, A, M Gott, L Jones and M Sidell (eds), *Health and Well-Being: A Reader*. Basingstoke: Macmillan, 55–67.

Armstrong, D (2003). Social theorising about health and illness. In Albrecht, GL, R Fitzpatrick and SC Scrimshaw (eds), *The Handbook of Social Studies in Health and Medicine*. London: Sage, 24–35.

Asthana, A (2006). Leading head attacks 'size zero' culture. *Observer*, 19 November.

Audi, R (2004). *The Good in the Right: A Theory of Intrinsic Value*. Princeton, NJ: Princeton University Press.

BBC News (2007). Trust overturns its obesity policy. www.news.bbc.co.uk (last accessed 28 April 2008).

BBC News (2008). Anti-depressant advice 'misleading'. www.news.bbc.co.uk (last accessed 28 April 2008).

Baird-Callicott, J (2005). The intrinsic value of nature in public policy: the case of the Endangered Species Act. In Cohen, AI and C Heath-Wellman (eds), *Contemporary Debates in Applied Ethics*. Malden, MA: Blackwell, 279–97.

Beauchamp, TL and JF Childress (2001). *Principles of Biomedical Ethics* (Fifth Edition). New York: Oxford University Press.

Becker, HS, B Geer, EC Hughes and AL Strauss (1977). *Boys in White: Student Culture in Medical School*. New Brunswick, NJ: Transaction Books.

Benatar, S and P Singer (2000). A new look at international research ethics. *British Medical Journal*, 321, 824–6.

Berlin, I (2002). Two concepts of liberty. In H Hardy (ed.), *Isaiah Berlin: Liberty*. New York: Oxford University Press, 166–217.

Blastland, M (2006). Essay. *New Statesman*, 17 April, 32–5.

Blastland, M (2007). *Joe: The Only Boy in the World*. London: Profile.

Boden, R (2004). *Sed quis custodiet ipsos custodies?* Governmentality, corporate governance and ethics. Paper presented to the Corporate Governance and Ethics Conference, Macquarie Graduate School of Management, Sydney, Australia, 28–30 June.

Bogdanor, V et al. (2007). In search of British values. *Prospect*, October, 22–6.

Bonnett, A (2001). *How to Argue*. Harlow: Pearson Education.

Bower, P, S Gilbody, D Richards, J Fletcher and A Sutton (2006). Collaborative care for depression in primary care: making sense of a complex intervention: systematic review and meta-regression. *British Journal of Psychiatry*, 189, 6, 484–93.

Bowles, W, M Collingridge, S Curry and B Valentine (2006). *Ethical Practice in Social Work*. Maidenhead: Open University Press.

Bradshaw, PL and G Bradshaw (2004). *Health Policy for Health Care Professionals*. London: Sage.

British Association of Social Workers (BASW) (2002). *The Code of Ethics for Social Work*. www.bassw.co.uk (last accessed 5 May 2008).

Broom, A and E Willis (2007). Competing paradigms and health research. In Saks, M and J Allsop (eds), *Researching Health*. London: Sage, 16–31.

Buchanan, AE (1984). The right to a decent minimum of health care. *Philosophy and Public Affairs*, 13, 1, 55–78.

Burleigh, M (2001). *The Third Reich: A New History*. London: Pan Macmillan.

Buruma, I (2007). *Murder in Amsterdam: The Death of Theo Van Gogh and the Limits of Tolerance*. London: Atlantic Books.

Campbell, AV (1990). Education or indoctrination: the issue of autonomy in health education. In Doxiadis, S (ed.), *Ethics in Health Education*. Chichester: Wiley, 15–28.

Campbell, D (2006). Junk food ads face ban in youth magazines. *Observer*, 19 November.

Carr, D (2003). *Making Sense of Education*. Abingdon: Routledge.

Central Office for Research Ethics Committees (COREC) (2001). *Governance Arrangements for NHS Research Ethics Committees*. London: COREC.

Clouder, L (2003). Becoming professional: exploring the complexities of professional socialisation in health and social care. *Learning in Health and Social Care*, 2, 4, 213–22.

Cohen, P (2006). Instant expert: genetics. *New Scientist*, 4 September. www.newscientist.com (last accessed 25 May 2008).

College of Occupational Therapy (2001). *Code of Ethics and Professional Conduct for Occupational Therapists*. London: College of Occupational Therapy.

Cookson, R and P Donlan (2000). Principles of justice in health care rationing. *Journal of Medical Ethics*, 26, 323–29.

Cooter, R (2000). The ethical body. In Cooter, R and J Pickstone (eds), *Medicine in the 20th Century*. London: Harwood Academic Publishers, 451–68.

Cottingham, J (ed.) (2008). *Western Philosophy: An Anthology*. Oxford: Blackwell.

Cox, BD et al. (1987). *The Health and Lifestyle Survey: Preliminary Report*. Cambridge: The Health Promotion Research Trust.

Cribb, A (2005). *Health and the Good Society: Setting Bioethics in its Social Context*. Oxford: Oxford University Press.

Cribb, A and S Bignold (1999). Towards the reflexive medical school: the hidden curriculum and medical education research. *Studies in Higher Education* 24, 2, 195–209.

Cribb, A and P Duncan (2002). *Health Promotion and Professional Ethics*. Oxford: Blackwell Science.

Dawson, AJ (1994). Professional codes of practice and ethical conduct. *Journal of Applied Philosophy*, 11, 2, 145–53.

Deacon, A (2002). *Perspectives on Welfare*. Buckingham: Open University Press.

Department of Health (1997). *The Nurses, Midwives and Health Visitors Act 1997*. London: HMSO.

Department of Health (2004). *Choosing Health*. London: HMSO.

Department of Health (2006). *Health Act 2006*. London: HMSO.

Department of Health and Social Services (1977). *The National Health Service Act 1977*. London: HMSO.

Dougherty, CJ (1993). Bad faith and victim-blaming: the limits of health promotion. *Health Care Analysis*, 1, 111–19.

Douglas, J, S Earle, S Handsley, C Lloyd, and S Spurr (eds) (2007). *A Reader in Promoting Public Health: Challenge and Controversy*. Milton Keynes/London: The Open University/Sage.

Downie, RS, C Tannahill and A Tannahill (1996). *Health Promotion: Models and Values* (Second Edition). Oxford: Oxford University Press.

Duncan, P (2004). Dispute, dissent and the place of health promotion in a 'disrupted tradition' of health improvement. *Public Understanding of Science*, 13, 2, 177–90.

Duncan, P (2007). *Critical Perspectives on Health*. Basingstoke: Palgrave Macmillan.

Duncan, P (2008). Ethics and law and health. In Naidoo, J and J Wills (eds), *Health Studies: An Introduction*. Basingstoke: Palgrave Macmillan, 345–71.

Duncan, P and A Cribb (1996). Helping people change: an ethical approach? *Health Education Research*, 11, 3, 339–48.

Dworkin, R (1995). *Life's Dominion: An Argument about Abortion and Euthanasia*. London: HarperCollins.

Dyer, C (2006). GP questioned over journey to suicide clinic. *Guardian*, 31 January.

Earle, S (2007). Exploring health. In Earle, S, CE Lloyd, M Sidel and S Spurr (eds), *Theory and Research in Promoting Public Health*. London: Sage, 37–65.

Earle, S, CE Lloyd, M Sidell and S Spurr (eds) (2007). *Theory and Research in Promoting Public Health*. London: Sage.

Easton, D (1953). *The Political System*. New York: Alfred A Knopf.

Edgar, A (1994). The value of codes of conduct. In Hunt, G (ed.), *Ethical Issues in Nursing*. London: Routledge, 148–63.

Edwards, SD (2001). *Philosophy of Nursing: An Introduction*. Basingstoke: Palgrave Macmillan.

Englehardt Jr, HT and KW Wildes (1994). The four principles of health care ethics: why a libertarian interpretation is unavoidable. In Gillon, R and A Lloyd (eds), *Principles of Health Care Ethics*. Chichester: Wiley, 135–47.

Family Heart Study Group (1994). Randomised controlled trial evaluating cardiovascular screening and intervention in general practice: principal results of the British Family Heart Study. *British Medical Journal*, 308, 313–20.

Fitzpatrick, M (2001). *The Tyranny of Health: Doctors and the Regulation of Lifestyle*. London: Routledge.

Freedom to Care (2008). Charge Nurse Graham Pink blows whistle on nurse under-staffing. www.freedomtocare.org (last accessed 16 July 2008).

Gillon, R (1990). *Philosophical Medical Ethics*. Chichester: Wiley.

Gillon, R (1994). Medical ethics: four principles plus attention to scope. *British Medical Journal*, 309, 184–8.

Gillon, R and A Lloyd (eds) (1994). *Principles of Health care Ethics*. Chichester: Wiley.

Glover, J (1977). *Causing Death and Saving Lives*. Harmondsworth: Penguin.

Glover, J (2006). *Choosing Children: The Ethical Dilemmas of Genetic Intervention*. Oxford: Oxford University Press.

Gorovitz, S (1985). *Doctors' Dilemmas: Moral Conflict and Medical Care*. New York: Oxford University Press.

Grayling, AC (2003). *What is Good? The Search for the Right Way to Live*. London: Wiedenfeld and Nicolson.

Guardian (2002). Dianne Pretty loses right to die case. *Guardian*, 29 April.

Haldane, JJ (1986). 'Medical ethics' – an alternative approach. *Journal of Medical Ethics*, 12, 145–50.

Halper, E (2003). Ethics in film. *APA Newsletter*, 3, 1, 191–5.

Halstead, JM and MJ Reiss (2003). *Values in Sex Education: From Principles to Practice*. London: Routledge Falmer.

Ham, C (2004). *Health Policy in Britain* (Fifth Edition). Basingstoke: Palgrave Macmillan.

Harding, L (2005). Swiss hospital will be the first to allow assisted suicide. *Guardian Weekly*, 23 December.

Hardy, A (2001). *Health and Medicine in Britain since 1860*. Basinsgstoke: Palgrave.

Hare, RM (1994). Utilitarianism and deontological principles. In Gillon, R and A Lloyd (eds), *Principles of Health Care Ethics*. Chichester: Wiley, 149–57.

Hart, C (2004). *Nurses and Politics: The Impact of Power and Practice*. Basingstoke: Palgrave Macmillan.

Herzlich, C (1973). *Health and Illness*. New York: Academic Press.

Holliday, A (2002). *Doing and Writing Qualitative Research*. London: Sage.

House of Commons Health Committee (2006). *Smoking in Public Places: First Report of Session 2005–6* (Vol. 1). London: The Stationery Office.

Hoyle, E (1980). Professionalisation and deprofessionalisation in education. In Hoyle, E and J Megarry (eds), *World Yearbook of Education 1980*. London: Kogan Page, 42–56.

Illich, I (1977). *Limits to Medicine*. London: Pelican.

Imperial Cancer Research Fund Oxcheck Study Group (1995). Effectiveness of health checks conducted by nurses in primary care: final results of the Oxcheck study. *British Medical Journal*, 310, 1099–1104.

Jackson, J (2006). *Ethics in Medicine*. Cambridge: Polity Press.

Jonsen, AR (1998). *The Birth of Bioethics*. Oxford: Oxford University Press.

Kennedy, I (1981). *The Unmasking of Medicine*. London: George Allen and Unwin.

Kennedy, I (2001). *Inquiry into the Management and Care of Children Receiving Complex Heart Surgery at the Bristol Royal Infirmary* (The Kennedy Inquiry Report). Norwich: The Stationery Office.

Kitcher, P (1997). *The Lives to Come: The Genetic Revolution and Human Possibilities*. London: Penguin.

Koehn, D (1994). *The Ground of Professional Ethics*. London: Routledge.

Lacey, AR (1976). *A Dictionary of Philosophy*. London: Routledge and Kegan Paul.

Leith, P (2007). Interview. *Today*, 13 December. www.bbc.co.uk/radio4/today. (last accessed 25 July 2008).

Lucas, K and B Lloyd (2005). *Health Promotion: Evidence and Experience*. London: Sage.

Macdonald, TH (2006). *Health, Trade and Human Rights*. Oxford: Radcliffe.

Macintyre, A (1985). *After Virtue: A Study in Moral Theory* (Second Edition). London: Duckworth.

Mackie, JL (1977). *Ethics: Inventing Right and Wrong*. Harmondsworth: Penguin.

Macnaughton, J (2007). Literature and the 'good doctor' in Ian McEwan's 'Saturday'. *Medical Humanities*, 33, 70–4.

Marshall, L and F Rowland (1998). *A Guide to Learning Independently* (Third Edition). Buckingham: Open University Press.

Marteau, TM (1989). Psychological costs of screening. *British Medical Journal*, 299, 527 (26 August).

Marteau TM (1990) Screening in practice: reducing the psychological costs. *British Medical Journal*, 301, 26–8.

McKeown, T (1976). *The Role of Medicine: Dream, Mirage or Nemesis*. London: Nuffield Provincial Hospitals Trust.

Meikle, J (2004). Doctors helping patients to die. *Guardian Unlimited*. www.guardian.co.uk (last accessed 30 November 2006).

Mill, JS (1962). *Utilitarianism and Other Writings* (edited by Mary Warnock). Glasgow: Fontana.

Mittlemark, MB (2007). Setting an ethical agenda for health promotion. *Health Promotion International*, 23, 1, 78–85.

National Health Service/Home Office (2008). *Alcohol: Know Your Limits*. www.knowyourlimits.gov.uk (last accessed 21 January 2008).

Neuberger, J (2005). *The Moral State We're In*. London: HarperCollins.

NHS Centre for Reviews and Dissemination (NHSCRD) (2002). *Effective Health Care Bulletin: The Prevention and Treatment of Childhood Obesity*. York: NHSCRD.

Nixon, J and P Sikes (2003). Introduction: reconceptualising the debate. In Sikes, P, J Nixon and W Carr (eds), *The Moral Foundations of Educational Research*. Maidenhead: Open University Press, 1–5.

Nixon, J, M Walker and P Clough (2003). Research as thoughtful practice. In Sikes, P, J Nixon and W Carr (eds), *The Moral Foundations of Educational Research*. Maidenhead: Open Uiversity Press, 86–104.

Nordenfelt, L (1993). On the nature and ethics of health promotion: an attempt at a systematic analysis. *Health Care Analysis*, 1, 121–30.

Nuffield Council on Bioethics (2005). *The Ethics of Research Related to Health Care in Developing Countries*. London: Nuffield Council on Bioethics.

Nursing and Midwifery Council (2004). *The NMC Code of Professional Conduct, Standards for Conduct, Performance and Ethics*. London: Nursing and Midwifery Council.

Oliver, P (2003). *The Student's Guide to Research Ethics*. Maidenhead: Open University Press.

Oxford University Press (1983). *The Oxford Paperback Dictionary* (Second Edition). Oxford: Oxford University Press.

Palmer, GR and MT Ho (2008). *Health Economics: A Critical and Global Analysis*. Basingstoke: Palgrave Macmillan.

Paton, HJ (1948). *The Moral L aw*. London: Hutchinson.

Peters, RS (1973). Aims of education: a conceptual enquiry. In Peters, RS (ed.), *The Philosophy of Education*. Oxford: Oxford University Press, 11–29.

Plant, R (1989). *Can There Be a Right to Health Care?* Southampton: Institute for Health Policy Studies.

Plant, R (2002). Can there be a right to a basic income? Paper presented to the BIEN Ninth International Congress, Geneva, Switzerland, 12–14 September.

Porter, R (1999). *The Greatest Benefit to Mankind*. London: HarperCollins.

Porter, S (1995). *Nursing's Relationship with Medicine: A Critical Realist Ethnography*. Aldershot: Avebury.

Randall, F and RS Downie (2006). *The Philosophy of Palliative Care: Critique and Reconstruction*. Oxford: Oxford University Press.

Rawson, D (1994). Willpower and authentic choice in stopping smoking. *Health Care Analysis*, 2, 201–5.

Reich, WT (1995). *The Encyclopaedia of Bioethics*. New York: Simon & Schuster.

Revill, J (2006a). Patients' lives being left at mercy of abusive nurses. *Observer*, 25 June.

Revill, J (2006b). NHS must pay for fat children to get surgery. *Observer*, 19 November.

Royal College of Nursing (2007). *Blowing the Whistle: Information for Nurses*. London: Royal College of Nursing.

Russell, B (1979). *A History of Western Philosophy*. London: Unwin Paperbacks.

Ryan, C (2006). IVF 'good for British economy'. http://news.bbc.co.uk (last accessed 12 May 2008).

Saks, M and J Allsop (eds) (2007). *Researching Health: Qualitative, Quantitative and Mixed Methods*. London: Sage.

Scadding, JG (1988). Health and disease: what can medicine do for philosophy? *Journal of Medical Ethics*, 14, 118–24.

Seedhouse, D (1998). *Ethics: The Heart of Health Care* (Second Edition). Chichester: Wiley.

Seedhouse, D (2001). *Health: The Foundations for Achievement* (Second Edition). Chichester: Wiley.

Skrabanek, P and J McCormick (1989). *Follies and Fallacies in Medicine*. Glasgow: The Tarragon Press.

Smart, JJC (1967). Extreme and restricted utilitarianism. In Foot, P (ed.), *Theories of Ethics*. Oxford: Oxford University Press, 171–83.

Smith, J (2002). *First Report: Death Disguised* (The Shipman Inquiry Report). London: The Stationery Office.

Smith, J (2003). *Second Report: The Police Investigation* (The Shipman Inquiry Report). London: The Stationery Office.

Sprague, E (1978). *Metaphysical Thinking*. New York: Oxford University Press.

Stanley, N and J Manthorpe (2004). The inquiry as Janus. In Stanley, N and J Manthorpe (eds), *The Age of the Inquiry: Learning and Blaming in Health and Social Care*. London: Routledge, 1–16.

Stohr, K (2006). Contemporary virtue ethics. *Philosophy Compass*, 1, 1, 22–7.

Sweney, M (2007). MPs seek tougher junk food ad ban. *Guardian*, 6 February.

Tate, S (2004). Using critical reflection as a teaching tool. In Tate, S and M Sills (eds), *The Development of Critical Reflection in the Health Professions*. London: Higher Education Academy Health Sciences and Practice Subject Centre, 8–17.

Tate, S and M Sills (eds) (2004). *The Development of Critical Reflection in the Health Professions*. London: Higher Education Academy Health Sciences and Practice Subject Centre.

Thomas, K (1997). Health and morality in early modern England. In Brandt, AM and P Rozin (eds), *Morality and Health*. New York: Routledge, 15–34.

Tomes, N (1997). Moralizing the microbe: the germ theory and the moral construction of behaviour in the late nineteenth-century antituberculosis movement. In Brandt, AM and P Rozin (eds), *Morality and Health*. New York: Routledge, 271–96.

Tones, K and J Green (2004). *Health Promotion: Planning and Strategies*. London: Sage.

Townsend, P, N Davidson and M Whitehead (1988). *Inequalities in Health*. London: Penguin.

Tudor Hart, J (1971). The inverse care law. *Lancet*, 27 February, 405–12.

Turner, BS (2003). The history of the changing concepts of health and illness: outline of a general model of illness categories. In Albrecht, GL, R Fitzpatrick and SC Scrimshaw (eds), *The Handbook of Social Studies in Health and Medicine*. London: Sage, 9–23.

Warburton, N (1999). *Philosophy: The Basics* (Third Edition). London: Routledge.

Warburton, N (2007). *Thinking from A to Z* (Third Edition). Abingdon: Routledge.

Wheelwright, S and S Baron-Cohen (2001). The link between autism and skills such as engineering, math, physics and computing: a reply to Jarrold and Routh. *Autism*, 5, 223–7.

Wikler, DI (1978). Persuasion and coercion for health: ethical issues in government efforts to change lifestyles. *Millbank Memorial Fund Quarterly/Health and Society*, 56, 3, 303–8.

Wikler, DI (1987). Who should be blamed for being sick? *Health Education Quarterly*, 14, 1, 11–25.

Wilkinson, RG (1996). *Unhealthy Societies: The Afflictions of Inequality*. London: Routledge.

Wilkinson, RG (2005). *The Impact of Inequality*. Abingdon: Routledge.

Williams, B (2002). *Truth and Truthfulness*. Princeton, NJ: Princeton University Press.

Williams, R (1983). Concepts of health: an analysis of lay logic. *Sociology*, 17, 2, 185–204.

Wilson, M (1975). *Health is for People*. London: Darton, Longman and Todd.

Woodward, W (2006). Lords vote to block assisted suicide bill for terminally ill. *Guardian Unlimited*. www.guardian.co.uk (last accessed 30 November 2006).

Worrall, J (2007). Evidence in medicine and evidence-based medicine. *Philosophy Compass*, November.

Wright, K (2007). Human rights in primary care. In Baruma, D and J Spicer (eds), *Primary Care Ethics*. Oxford: Radcliffe, 55–69.

INDEX